Alexandra David

RENAL DIET COOKBOOK FOR BEGINNERS

A Collection of 200 Delicious and Simple Recipes to Help You Manage Your Kidneys and Optimize Your Health Quickly and Easily (Updated for 2020/2021)

© Copyright 2020 - All rights reserved.

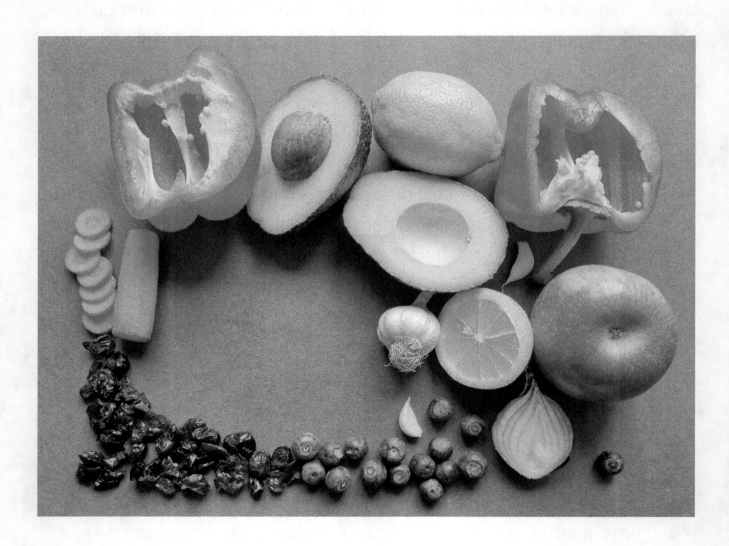

TABLE OF CONTENTS

CHAPTER 6: VEGAN AND VEGETABLES . 88

CHAPTER 7: SNACKS 102

CHAPTER 8: SOUPS AND SALADS 122

CHAPTER 9: DESSERT RECIPES 148

CONCLUSION 170

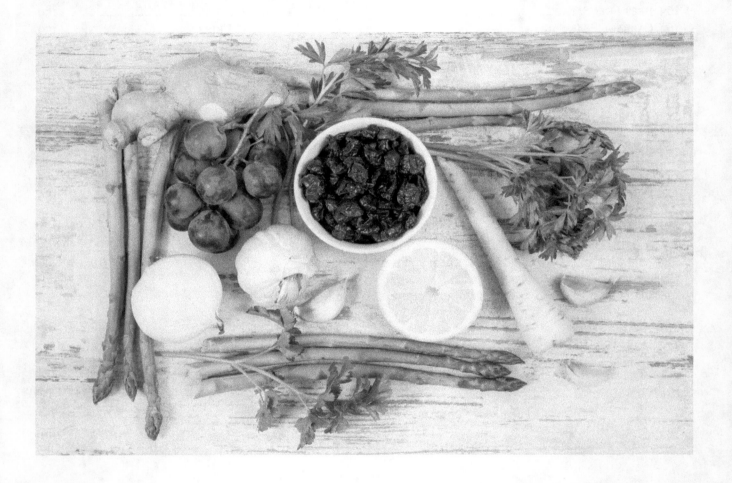

Introduction

Maintaining an easy renal diet isn't always easy. Whether you want to provide healthy meals and snacks for your busy life . . . or stay fit to feel great, look good, and reduce your chances of a health issue . . . or simply sort through the latest nutrition news to find sound advice . . . this book is for you. This book reflects the latest renal diet guide; it's all about prevention first—and your overall food and beverage choices over time, it's not a single food, meal, or snack diet.

Healthy eating advice for every renal diet patient—from feeding an infant, child, or teen, to the different food and nutrition needs of both women and men, and the special challenges of aging.

Advice for common renal diet health issues—promoting gut health, a healthy weight, and immunity; preventing, slowing, and dealing with heart disease, cancer, diabetes, among others; managing a food allergy, celiac disease, or lactose intolerance; and addressing many other health issues.

First, it's important to clarify that sodium is not a synonym for salt, as many people believe. Salt is just a compound of sodium and chloride. On the other hand, sodium is a mineral naturally present in many foods and important for body functions. In addition to potassium and chloride, sodium is an electrolyte, which means it helps control fluid levels in cells and tissues.

Sodium helps maintain blood pressure, regulates nerve function and muscle contraction, controls acid-base balance in the blood, among other things.

However, excessive levels of sodium are harmful to patients with kidney disease due to the fact these organs are unable to eliminate sodium and fluids from the body in an adequate manner.

As a result, fluid and sodium start accumulating and may cause a number of problems such as increased thirst, edema, hypertension, heart failure, and shortness of breath.

Phosphorus is a mineral required for the maintenance and development of bones. This mineral also participates in the development of connective tissues, takes part in muscle movement, and so much more. Damaged kidneys don't remove excess phosphorus from the body. In turn, levels of this mineral accumulate and impair calcium balance, thus causing weak bones and calcium deposits in blood vessels.

Potassium is an important mineral that participates in many functions, including muscle function, and it helps promote a healthy heartbeat. Like sodium, potassium is also necessary for fluid and electrolyte balance. While potassium is needed for our health, patients with kidney disease do need to reduce the intake of this mineral. The reason is simple; when kidneys are damaged, they are not able to eliminate excess potassium out of the body. This causes a buildup of potassium and leads to other problems such as muscle weakness, heart attack, slow pulse, and and irregular heartbeat.

Protein is one of the most important nutrients we need to consume on a daily basis. Generally speaking, protein is not a problem for people with healthy kidneys because it is eliminated out of the body with the help of renal proteins and filtering units. But people with kidney disease need to be cautious about how much protein they consume because their body doesn't remove this nutrient properly.

CHAPTER 1:

What Is Kidney Disease

The kidneys are a couple of fist-sized organs situated at the bottom of the rib restrain. On each side of the backbone, there is one kidney.

Both of the kidneys are basic to having a healthy body. They are the most part liable for separating waste items, excess water, and different polluting impurities from our body. These impurities are kept in the bladder and then can be removed through the urine. Straightly, the kidneys have different levels like potassium or salt. They create hormones that control the BP and the creation of red blood cells. The kidneys even activate a type of vitamin D that enables the body to retain calcium.

Kidney disease influences roughly 26 million American adults. It happens when your kidneys become damaged and cannot perform their functions properly. The damage might be brought about by diabetes, blood pressure and different other chronic (long term) conditions. Kidney disease can lead to other medical issues, including weakness of bones, nerve harm, and lack of healthy sustenance.

If the kidney disease gets much worse after some time, your kidneys may quit working totally. This implies that dialysis needed to do the purpose of the kidneys. It is a cure that channels and filters the blood utilizing a machine. It cannot fix kidney disease. However, it can draw out your life.

Stages of CKD

Stage 1

At stage one, the functions of the kidneys are still normal and patients may not notice any obvious symptoms. But protein can be noticed in patients' urine if tested. The estimated glomerular filtration rate (GFR) of the kidneys at stage one is 90 ml per minute or above. This is similar to GFR of a healthy kidney.

Stage 2

Stage two chronic kidney disease (CKD) characterizes a mild decrease in kidney functions. At this point, a little rise in the level of creatinine in the blood can be noticed if the patient is tested. The estimated glomerular filtration rate (GFR) of the kidney in stage two is around 60 to 89 ml per minute.

Stage 3

Stage 3 is often referred to as the middle stage of chronic kidney disease (CKD). It is the most common category of chronic kidney disease. At stage 3, there is a moderate decrease in kidney functions and patients must have started to sense some complications of chronic kidney disease. These complications include anemia, high blood pressure, bone weakness and fatigue.

Stage 4

At stage four, the functions of the kidney will have decreased immensely and the patient will be faced with a lot of negative health conditions associated with chronic kidney disease (CKD). This stage is associated with severity. At this stage, doctors will already be planning for dialysis or kidney transplant. The estimated glomerular filtration rate (GFR) in stage four is around 15 to 29 ml per minute.

Stage 5

Stage five is the last stage of chronic kidney disease. This is the stage where the kidneys finally fail. The estimated glomerular filtration rate (GFR) is below 15 ml per minute. The kidneys may still be able to function a bit but the level of the kidney function at this stage will not be enough to keep the patient alive. At stage five the patient will need dialysis or kidney transplant to survive.

Eating Right with Chronic Kidney Disease

Particular foods should be limited if you have chronic kidney disease. There are also some foods that you could put in your diet that may help curb symptoms and avoid dialysis. If you are already on dialysis, follow the eating program provided by your physician. Before beginning any kidney disease diet, check with your healthcare professional.

It can be challenging deciding what and how to eat correctly with this disease. There are lots of foods that will need to be removed or restricted.

But, you will also need to eat enough calories to maintain a decent energy level and stay healthy. A healthy weight has to be maintained. You do not want to lose weight since this will put you at risk for other health problems or different diseases.

Please remember to discuss your diet plans completely with your healthcare professional. Additionally, it would be advantageous to sit down and talk with a nurse or dietitian to assist with healthy choices while on the kidney disorder diet.

As a general rule, sufferers of chronic kidney disease have to restrict their intake of phosphorus and the mineral potassium. Sodium and protein will have to be consumed at carefully measured levels, and you will want to track how much liquids you ingest.

About 5 to 7 ounces a day of high protein foods may be eaten. Protein is a tricky one as you will need enough to possess energy and fight disease, but too much can strain the kidneys. Being educated about protein foods will help in tracking them closely.

Retention can cause issues for CKD sufferers. When the kidneys are in distress, it will not be easy for them to manage an excessive amount of salt in the body—they might have to work harder to eliminate excess sodium.

Limiting sodium has additional advantages like helping combat fluid retention, a problem with this disease.

Another thing to monitor closely when observing a kidney disorder diet is fluid ingestion. Talk to your doctor or dietitian; monitoring will allow you to maintain a safe quantity of fluids.

Always check with your doctor before making any changes to dieting customs or strategies. Read labels to be familiar with ingredients that are included. Eating a healthy diet can help prevent further kidney damage.

The Most Common Causes of Kidney Disease

Renal disease, according to experts, requires early diagnosis and targeted treatment to prevent or delay both a condition of acute or chronic renal failure and the appearance of cardiovascular complications to which it is often associated.

In fact, hypertension and diabetes, not adequately controlled by drug therapy, prostatic hypertrophy, kidney stones, or bulky tumors can promote onset as they reduce the normal flow of urine, increase the pressure inside the kidneys and limit functionality.

Or the kidney damage can be determined by inflammatory processes (pyelonephritis, glomerulonephritis) or by the formation of cysts inside the kidneys (polycystic kidney disease) or by the chronic use of some drugs, alcohol, and drugs consumed in excess.

A fundamental role in alleviating the work of the already compromised kidneys is carried out by the diet which is, therefore, the first prevention.

It must be studied with an expert nutritionist or a nephrologist in order to maintain or reach an ideal weight on the one hand, and on the other to reduce the intake of sodium (salt), and the consequent control of blood pressure, and/or other substances (minerals), without creating malnutrition or nutritional deficiencies. Particular attention should also be paid to cholesterol, triglycerides and blood sugar levels.

Understanding what causes kidney failure goes a long way to deciding just what kind of treatment you should focus on. The most important factor that you should focus on is, of course, your diet. But as you focus on your diet, make sure that you are following your doctor's instructions, in the event of other complications. Let us look at a few of the common causes of kidney diseases.

Diabetes

We do know that diabetes is one of the leading causes of CKD. But we have yet to understand in detail why and how it can cause so much harm to the kidneys.

Time for a crash course in diabetes. What many may already know is that diabetes affects our body's insulin production rate. But what many may not know is the extent of damage that diabetes can cause to the kidneys.

High Blood Pressure

An important thing to remember here is that high blood pressure can be both a cause and symptom of CKD, similar to the case of diabetes.

So, what exactly is blood pressure? People often throw the term around, but they are unable to pinpoint exactly what happens when the pressure in the blood increases.

Autoimmune Diseases

IgA nephropathy and lupus are two examples of autoimmune diseases that can lead to kidney diseases. But just what exactly are autoimmune diseases?

They are conditions where your immune system perceives your body as a threat and begins to attack it.

We all know that the immune system is like the defense force of our body. It is responsible for guiding the soldiers of our body, known as white blood cells, or WBCs. The immune system is responsible for fighting against foreign materials, such as viruses and bacteria. When the system senses these foreign bodies, various fighter cells, including the WBCs, are deployed in order to combat the threat.

Typically, your immune system is a self-learning system. This means that it is capable of understanding the threat and memorizing its features, behaviors, and attack patterns. This is an important capability of the immune system since it allows the system to differentiate between our own cells and foreign cells. But when you have an autoimmune disease, your immune system suddenly considers certain parts of your body, such as your skin or joints, as foreign. It then proceeds to create antibodies that begin to attack these parts.

CHAPTER 2:

What Is the Renal Diet?

A renal diet is low in sodium, phosphorus, and protein. A renal diet also emphasizes how important it is to consume high-quality protein and generally limit fluid intake. Some patients may also need to limit potassium and calcium. The body of each person is different and therefore, each patient must work with a renal dietician to develop a diet that meets the needs of the patient.

Protein: Proteins are not a problem for healthy kidneys. Normally, the proteins are taken up and waste is produced, which in turn is filtered by kidney nephrons.

Then the waste becomes urine with the help of additional kidney proteins. In contrast, damaged kidneys do not eliminate protein waste and accumulate in the blood. Sufficient protein intake is difficult in patients with chronic renal failure because the amount varies with each stage of the disease. Proteins are crucial for maintaining tissue and other bodily functions. Therefore, it is important to consume the amount that your renal nephrologist or nutritionist recommends for each stage of the disease.

Fiber: Dietary fiber is defined as the carbohydrate component that cannot be digested by enzymes in the human small intestine. Fiber provides a structure for plant cells. It occurs in fruits, vegetables, cereals, legumes, and nuts. Unlike fats, carbohydrates, and proteins, fibers cannot be broken down or absorbed by the digestive system.

You need integration and good habits

Learning to integrate "diet" directions with traditional ones can make the difference on the success of the nutritional treatment. The point is to initially dedicate some time to the evaluation of the favorite recipes and to the selection of the ingredients.

Small modifications of traditional dishes, as long as they are actually tested, can be pleasant for the whole family.

Even a person with chronic kidney disease can afford a plate of lasagna or cannelloni. Maybe preparing them with vegetables and vegetable béchamel sauce. Even vegetable soufflé, pizza or vegetable pies, peppers or baked pasta are not taboo: they can be, if properly prepared, foods low in sodium and protein, but tasty for all members of the family.

Today, even women, once the sole owner of the kitchen, are often away from home. Their role is delegated to others, to the food industry, or to restaurants. Sometimes it can be difficult to combine kidney failure and nutrition, and other health issues, with professional and relationship life.

However, one must not give up one's recurrences, convivial meetings, or work. By adopting some tricks, even a super-woman can adopt a lifestyle suitable for the proper management of her kidney function.

In addition to the choice of food, it is important to combine tools, weekly menus and cooking directions appropriately, so as to enhance the taste of the food and the variety. For example, you can boil vegetables in water to reduce the potassium content and put them in the oven or pan with the addition of aromatic herbs, so as to have dishes low in sodium. The elaboration of a weekly menu thinking of the family and shared with the trusted dietician can be a valid help to solve the problem of boredom in the kitchen. This enemy of good food can be eradicated! Coordination and collaboration between family members and therapists is enough to manage disease, kidney failure and nutrition.

Purifying the kidneys has been a way to avoid the formation of calcium deposits in these two important organs since ancient times. Calcium accumulations can sometimes increase the size of a kidney stone, causing severe pain. The kidneys, in fact, are very delicate organs that filter blood. Therefore, it is good to perform a regular "cleaning," both through the diet and through the use of an herbal program. Herbal cleansing is, in fact, aimed at gently dissolving calcium deposits and other elements that can accumulate in the kidneys.

Foods that help maintain high potassium levels are particularly suitable for the kidneys. Bananas, nuts and grape juice are recommended, as are beans and dark green leafy vegetables. In fact, vegetables are rich in nutrients, including calcium, which helps to reduce the risk of developing kidney stones, keeping oxalate levels low. Cabbage, for example, can be eaten raw or cooked, you can also make fruit juices, using a blender or an extractor. A serving of two cups of cabbage has between 15 and 20% of the recommended daily calcium intake for men and adult women, with 201 milligrams of calcium per serving. There are many dietary protocols based on herbs that have been studied to purify the kidneys. Some of these are very delicate, others have a more aggressive approach and require a shorter duration, in any case, they are protocols to adapt subjectively and always with caution.

The Connection Between Diet and Kidney Disease

There is a distinct connection between the health and function of our kidneys and the way we eat. How we eat and the foods we choose make a significant impact on how well we feel and our overall wellbeing. Making changes to your diet is often necessary to guard against medical conditions, and while eating well can treat existing conditions, healthy food choices can also help prevent many other conditions from developing—including kidney disease.

When we make changes on our diet, we often focus on the restrictions or foods we should avoid. While this is important, it's also vital to learn about the foods and nutrients we need in order to maintain good health and prevent disease. Consider the related conditions that contribute to high blood pressure and type 2 diabetes, and the dietary changes often suggested to treat and, in some successful cases, reverse the damage of these conditions. Dietary changes for the treatment and prevention of disease often focus on limiting salt, sugar, and Tran's fats from our food choices, while increasing minerals, protein, and fiber, among other beneficial nutrients. The renal diet also focuses on eliminating, or at least limiting, the consumption of various ingredients to aid our kidneys to function better and to prevent further damage from occurring.

What to Eat and What to Avoid in Renal Diet

What to Avoid

- Some cereals: Oatmeal, whole wheat grains, cookies, pancakes, waffles, muffins, biscuits, pretzels.

- Some meats and fish: Deli meats, salmon, sardines, organ meats.

- Drinks to avoid: Colas, soft drinks.

- Avoid foods high in potassium: Bananas, avocados, most fish, potatoes, spinach, artichokes, dates, oranges.

- Avoid foods high in phosphorous: Processed cheese, red meat, fast food, milk, colas, and canned fish.

- Avoid foods high in sodium: Canned foods, processed foods, sauces, condiments, soy sauce, seasonings and salt added to your foods, avoid packaged or deli meats and control your portions well.

- Limit Your Intake of The Following Foods: Peanut butter, nuts in general, beans, seeds, butter or margarine.

What to Eat

- Drinks: you can favor the following drinks in your renal diet: some water, citrus based juices, wine, cranberry juice. Please consult with your doctor to know the right amount of fluids you should drink, depending on your kidneys conditions and the treatments you are going under. Don't forget to include the liquids included in soups or other liquid dishes.

- Eat Plenty of Vegetables: Corn, carrot, cabbage peas, eggplants, celery, lettuce, asparagus, bean sprouts, red bell peppers, onions, garlic, and cauliflower.

- Choose Low Sugar Fruits: Cranberries, apples, cherries, blackberries, blueberries, mangoes, pears, peaches, grapes.

- Others Privilege: olive oil, eggs, lean meats like poultry, beef, pork, coriander, ginger.

CHAPTER 3:

Breakfast Recipes

1. Buttermilk Pancakes

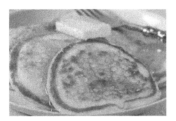

Preparation Time: 10 minutes

Cooking Time: 20 minutes

Servings: 2

Ingredients

- ½ cup almond flour

- ¼ teaspoon cream of tartar

- ½ teaspoons baking soda

- ½ tablespoons honey

- ½ cups low-fat buttermilk

- 1 egg

- ¼ tablespoon olive oil

Directions

1. Warm up a skillet on medium heat.

2. Combine dry ingredients in a large bowl. Add dry ingredients to buttermilk, oil and egg mixture. Use a whisk or spoon to blend the dry ingredients until they are completely moist. Use a teaspoon of olive oil to grease the skillet. Using a ⅓-cup measuring cup, scoop the pancake mixture on the skillet. Each pancake should spread to about 4 inches across. Leave about 2 inches between the pancakes for easy flipping. Flip pancakes using a spatula—do this when the bubbles on the top of the pancakes have mostly disappeared. Allow the other side to brown until the center no longer appears wet.

3. Move to a serving dish.

4. For a healthier twist, think of serving with fresh berries and a side of eggs.

Nutrition

- Calories: 124 Total Fat: 9.2g

- Saturated Fat: 1.1g

- Cholesterol: 42mg Sodium: 206mg

- Total Carbohydrate: 6.8g

- Protein: 5.4g Potassium: 94mg

- Phosphorus: 80mg

2. Egg Pockets

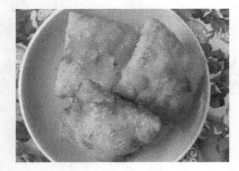

Preparation Time: 10 minutes

Cooking Time: 15 minutes

Servings: 2

Ingredients

- ¼ teaspoons dry yeast
- 1 cup warm water
- 1 tablespoon olive oil
- 1 tablespoon honey
- 1 garlic clove, minced
- ½ cup almond flour
- 1 egg
- ½ tablespoon cream cheese

Directions

1. Dissolve yeast in warm water. Stir in olive oil, honey, minced garlic, and almond flour to make a soft dough. Place in a greased bowl, cover and set aside. Let rest 5 minutes. Roll dough out to 1/2-inch thickness. Cut into 4 pieces. Scramble eggs and stir in cream cheese. Place egg mixture onto 1/2 of each piece of dough. Fold dough over, pinching edges, then cut top to vent.

2. Spray top of each pocket with oil

3. Bake at 350°F for 15 to 20 minutes, until light golden brown.

Nutrition

- Calories: 150 Total Fat: 12.1g
- Cholesterol: 42mg
- Sodium: 22mg
- Total Carbohydrate: 8.1g
- Protein: 4.9g Calcium: 41mg
- Iron: 1mg Potassium: 43mg
- Phosphorus: 35mg

3. Omelets with Vegetables

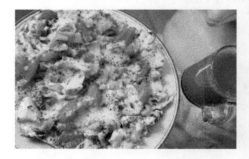

Preparation Time: 10 minutes

Cooking Time: 15 minutes

Servings: 2

Ingredients

- 1/8 cup zucchini, chopped
- 1/8 cup red bell pepper, chopped

- 1/8 cup kale, chopped

- 3 tablespoons green onion, chopped

- 2 tablespoons water

- 1/4 teaspoon dried dill

- 2 large egg whites

- 1 ounce low-fat sharp parmesan cheese, shredded

- ¼ tablespoon olive oil

Directions

1. Heat a small saucepan over medium-high heat. Coat pan with oil. Add bell pepper, zucchini, kale and onions to pan; sauté 4 minutes or until vegetables are crisp-tender. Remove from heat.

2. Heat a 10-inch non-stick skillet over medium-high heat. Combine water, pepper, dill, and egg whites in a bowl, stirring well with a whisk.

3. Coat pan with cooking spray. Pour egg mixture into pan; cook until edges begin to set (about 2 minutes). Gently lift the edges of the omelet with a spatula, tilting the pan to allow uncooked egg mixture to come into contact with the pan.

4. Spoon vegetable mixture onto half of omelet, sprinkle cheese over vegetable mixture. Loosen omelet with a spatula and fold in half. Cook 2 minutes more or until cheese melts. Carefully slide omelet onto a plate.

Nutrition

- Calories: 85

- Total Fat: 4g

- Saturated Fat: 2.5g

- Cholesterol: 10mg

- Sodium: 278mg

- Total Carbohydrate: 2.7g

- Protein: 9.5g

- Calcium: 196mg

- Iron: 0mg

- Potassium: 150mg

- Phosphorus: 118mg

4. Sausage Breakfast Sandwich

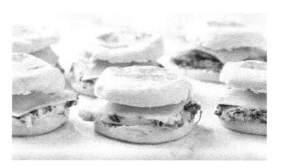

Preparation Time: 10 minutes

Cooking Time: 10 minutes

Servings: 2

Ingredients

- 1 egg

- 1 English muffin

- 1 turkey sausage patty

- 1 tablespoon shredded goat cheese

Directions

1. In a small skillet sprayed with non-stick cooking spray, pour egg and cook over medium-low heat. When egg appears almost cooked through, turn over with a spatula and cook an additional 30 seconds.

2. Toast English muffin.

3. Place turkey sausage patty on a plate, cover with a paper towel and cook in the microwave for 1 minute or the time recommended on the package.

4. Assemble cooked egg on English muffin (fold to fit muffin). Top with a sausage patty, then sharp goat cheese and remaining muffin half.

Nutrition

- Calories: 149 Total Fat: 5.5g

- Cholesterol: 104mg

- Sodium: 368mg

- Total Carbohydrate: 12.8g

- Protein: 11.4g Calcium: 84mg

- Potassium: 61mg Phosphorus: 58mg

5. Denver Omelets

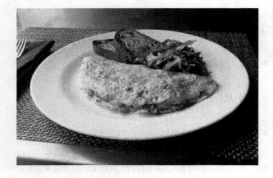

Prep Time: 4 minutes

Cook Time: 1 minute

Serving: 1

Ingredients

- 2 tablespoons almond butter

- ¼ cup onion, chopped

- ¼ cup green bell pepper, diced

- ¼ cup grape tomatoes halved

- 2 whole eggs

- ¼ cup ham, chopped

Directions

1. Take a skillet and place it over medium heat

2. Add butter and wait until the butter melts

3. Add onion and bell pepper and sauté for a few minutes

4. Take a bowl and whip eggs

5. Add the remaining ingredients and stir

6. Add sautéed onion and pepper, stir

7. Microwave the egg mix for 1 minute

8. Serve hot!

Nutrition

- Calories: 605 Fat: 46g

- Carbohydrates: 6g

- Protein: 39g

6. Garlic-Mint Scrambled Eggs

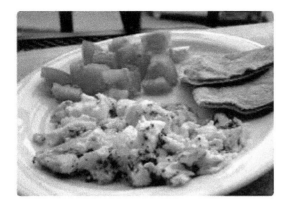

Preparation Time: 10 minutes

Cooking Time: 5 minutes

Servings: 2

Ingredients

- 4 large eggs
- ¼ cup soy milk
- 1 clove garlic, minced
- ¼ cup chopped fresh mint
- Pepper to taste
- 1 tablespoon olive oil
- ½ teaspoons freshly grated Parmesan cheese

Directions

1. Whisk together eggs, soy milk, and minced garlic until smooth; add mint and season to taste with pepper.

2. Heat olive oil in a non-stick skillet over medium heat. Pour in the egg mixture and cook to the desired degree of doneness, stirring constantly.

Nutrition

- Calories: 238
- Sodium: 192mg
- Protein:15.2g
- Potassium: 229mg
- Phosphorus: 107mg

7. Healthy Fruit Smoothie

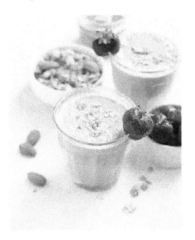

Preparation Time: 10 minutes

Cooking Time: 00 minutes

Servings: 2

Ingredients

- 1/3 cup fresh blueberries
- 1/3 cup fresh raspberries
- 4 large fresh strawberries, hulled
- 1/3 cup water
- 2/3 cup almond milk
- 2 tablespoons honey

Directions

1. Place the blueberries, raspberries, strawberries, water, milk, and honey into a blender. Cover, and puree until smooth. Pour into glasses to serve.

Nutrition

- Calories: 284

- Sodium: 15mg

- Protein: 2.6g

- Calcium: 26mg

- Potassium: 326mg

- Phosphorus: 117mg

8. Zucchini with Egg

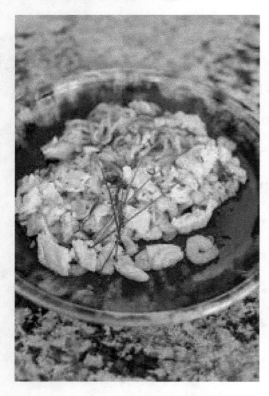

Preparation Time: 5 minutes

Cooking Time: 15 minutes

Servings: 2

Ingredients

- ½ tablespoons olive oil

- 2 large zucchini, cut into large chunks

- Ground black pepper to taste

- 2 large egg whites

Directions

1. Heat olive oil in a skillet over medium-high heat; sauté zucchini until tender, about 10 minutes. Season zucchini with black pepper.

2. Beat egg whites with a fork in a bowl; Pour eggs over zucchini; cook and stir until eggs are scrambled and no longer runny, about 5 minutes. Season zucchini and eggs with black pepper. Serve and enjoy.

Nutrition

- Calories: 99 Total

- Sodium: 66mg

- Protein: 7.5g

- Potassium: 91mg

- Phosphorus: 71mg

9. Green Slime Smoothie

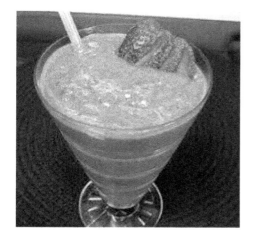

Preparation Time: 5 minutes

Cooking Time: 00 minutes

Servings: 2

Ingredients

- 1 cup kale
- 1 cup blueberries
- 1 tablespoon honey
- ¼ cup ice

Directions

1. Combine the kale, blueberries, honey, and ice in a blender. Blend until smooth.

2. Serve immediately.

Nutrition

- Calories: 90
- Sodium: 15mg
- Protein: 1.6g
- Calcium: 46mg

- Potassium: 226mg
- Phosphorus: 171mg

10. Baked Omelets Roll

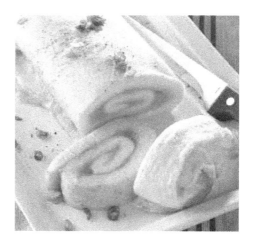

Preparation Time: 5 minutes

Cooking Time: 20 minutes

Servings: 2

Ingredients

- 2 egg whites
- ¼ cup soy milk
- 1/8 cup white flour
- 1/8 teaspoon ground black pepper
- ¼ cup shredded Cheddar cheese

Directions

1. Preheat oven to 450 degrees F. Lightly grease a 9x13-inch baking pan.

2. In a blender, combine egg whites, soy milk, almond flour, and pepper;

cover and process until smooth. Pour into prepared baking pan.

3. Bake in the preheated oven until set, about 20 minutes. Sprinkle with cheese.

4. Carefully loosen edges of omelet from pan. Starting from the short edge of the pan, carefully roll up omelet. Place omelet seam side down on a serving plate and cut into 4 equal-sized pieces

Nutrition

- Calories: 177 Total Fat: 13.1g

- Saturated Fat: 4.7g

- Sodium: 165mg

- Total Carbohydrate: 4g

- Protein. 11.6g Calcium: 148mg

- Potassium: 111mg

- Phosphorus: 91mg

11. Fresh Peaches Omelets

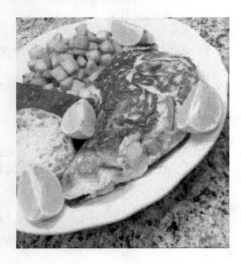

Preparation Time: 10 minutes

Cooking Time: 10 minutes

Servings: 2

Ingredients

- 1 egg white

- 1-1/2 tablespoons honey

- 1-1/2 tablespoons all-purpose flour

- 1/8 teaspoon baking powder

- 1 tablespoon almond milk

- ½ tablespoon lemon juice

- ½ teaspoon olive oil

- 1 large peach – peeled, cored and thinly sliced

- 1/8 teaspoon ground cinnamon

Directions

1. Preheat the oven to 350 degrees F.

2. In a medium bowl, whip egg white with an electric mixer until foamy. Sprinkle in honey, continuing to whip until stiff peaks form. In a separate bowl, stir together the flour, baking powder, and pepper. Mix in the almond milk and lemon juice until well blended, then fold in the egg whites using a rubber spatula or wooden spoon.

3. Heat the olive oil in a large cast-iron (or other ovenproof) skillet over medium heat. Spread the batter evenly in the pan. Layer the thinly sliced peaches over the batter and sprinkle with cinnamon.

4. Place the skillet in the oven, and bake for 10 minutes, or until the peaches are golden brown and glazed looking. Cut into wedges to serve.

Nutrition

- Calories: 113 Total Fat: 3.3g

- Saturated Fat: 1.8g

- Cholesterol: 0mg Sodium: 19mg

- Total Carbohydrate: 19.5g

- Dietary Fiber: 1.6g

- Total Sugars: 16.1g

- Protein: 3.1g

- Calcium: 19mg

- Potassium: 235mg

- Phosphorus: 131 mg

12. Caramelized French Toast

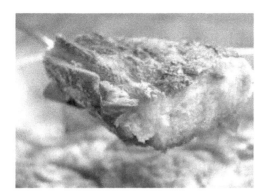

Preparation Time: 10 minutes

Cooking Time: 10 minutes

Servings: 2

Ingredients

- 1 tablespoon olive oil, divided

- 1 egg

- 1/8 cup almond milk

- 2 slices white bread

- ¼ cup brown sugar

- ¼ cup water

Directions

1. Heat ½ tablespoon of olive oil in a frying pan or skillet over medium-high heat.

2. Beat together egg, and almond milk. Dip bread one at a time into the egg mixture and fry until light brown and egg are cooked.

3. After all bread slices have been cooked and removed from the pan, add brown sugar to the pan. Stir until melted and sticky. Add water and stir. Place French toast in caramel sauce. Turn to coat, then remove from pan. Serve.

Nutrition

- Calories: 219 Total Fat: 13.1g

- Saturated Fat: 4.9g

- Cholesterol: 82mg Sodium: 100mg

- Total Carbohydrate: 23.3g

- Total Sugars: 18.7g Protein: 3.8g

- Calcium: 44mg Potassium: 102mg

- Phosphorus: 81mg

13. Egg Sandwich

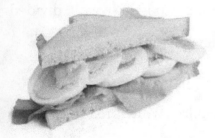

Preparation Time: 10 minutes

Cooking Time: 10 minutes

Servings: 2

Ingredients

- 2 egg whites
- 2 tablespoons almond milk
- 4 slices white bread
- Pepper to taste (optional)
- 2 slice American cheese

Directions

1. Crack the egg into a microwave-safe cereal bowl and whisk in the milk. Season with pepper. Cook in the microwave on 100% power for 1 to 2 minutes, or until cooked through. While the egg is cooking, toast the bread. Use a spoon to remove the cooked egg from the bowl and set it on one piece of toast. Top with a slice of cheese and the other piece of toast. Cook in the microwave until cheese is melted about 15 seconds

Nutrition

- Calories:169 Total Fat: 9.5g
- Saturated Fat: 6.4g
- Cholesterol: 17mg Sodium: 424mg
- Total Carbohydrate: 11.8g
- Total Sugars: 3.1g Protein: 9.2g
- Calcium: 152mg Potassium: 172mg
- Phosphorus: 100mg

14. Apple Tea Smoothie

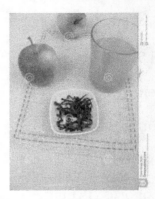

Preparation Time: 35 minutes

Cooking Time: 5 minutes

Servings: 2

Ingredients

- Unsweetened rice milk – 1 cup
- Tea bag – 1
- Apple – 1, peeled, cored, and chopped
- Ice – 2 cups

Directions

1. Heat the rice milk in a saucepan over low heat for 5 minutes, or until

steaming. Remove the milk from the heat and add to the tea bag to steep.

2. Let the milk cool in the refrigerator with the tea bag for 30 minutes. Then remove the tea bag, and squeeze gently to release all the flavor.

3. Place the milk, apple, and ice in a blender and blend until smooth.

4. Pour into 2 glasses and serve.

Nutrition

- Calories: 88 kcal Total Fat: 1 g

- Sodium: 47 mg Total Carbs: 19 g

- Protein: 1 g

15.   Blueberry-Pineapple Smoothie

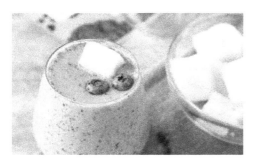

Preparation Time: 15 minutes

Cooking Time: 0 minutes

Servings: 2

Ingredients

- Frozen blueberries – 1 cup

- Pineapple chunks – ½ cup

- English cucumber – ½ cup

- Apple – ½

- Water – ½ cup

Directions

1. Put the pineapple, blueberries, cucumber, apple, and water in a blender and blend until thick and smooth.

2. Pour into 2 glasses and serve.

Nutrition

- Calories: 87kcal Total Fat: 1g

- Sodium: 3mg Total Carbs:22 g

16. Festive Berry Parfait

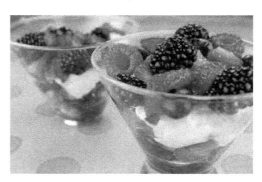

Preparation Time: 20 minutes

Cooking Time: 1 hour

Servings: 4

Ingredients

- Vanilla rice milk – 1 cup, at room temperature

- Plain cream cheese – ½ cup, room temp

- Granulated sugar - 1 tbsp.

- Ground cinnamon – ½ tsp.

- Crumbled meringue cookies – 1 cup

- Fresh blueberries – 2 cups

- Sliced fresh strawberries – 1 cup

Directions

1. In a small bowl, whisk together the milk, cream cheese, sugar, and cinnamon until smooth.

2. Into 4 (6-ounce) glasses, spoon ¼ cup of crumbled cookie in the bottom of each.

3. Spoon ¼ cup of the cream cheese mixture on top of the cookies.

4. Top the cream cheese with ¼ cup of the berries.

5. Repeat in each cup with the cookies, cream cheese mixture, and berries.

6. Chill in the refrigerator for 1 hour and serve.

Nutrition

- Calories: 243 kcal

- Total Fat: 1 g

- Sodium: 145 mg

- Total Carbs: 33 g

- Protein: 4 g

17. Simple Chia Porridge

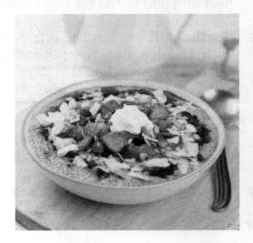

Preparation Time: 10 minutes

Cooking Time: 5-10 minutes

Serving: 2

Ingredients

- 1 tablespoon chia seeds

- 1 tablespoon ground flaxseed

- 1/3 cup coconut cream

- ½ cup of water

- 1 teaspoon vanilla extract

- 1 tablespoon almond butter

Direction

1. Add chia seeds, coconut cream, flaxseed, water and vanilla to a small pot

2. Stir and let it sit for 5 minutes

3. Add almond butter and place pot over low heat

4. Keep stirring as almond butter melts

5. Once the porridge is hot/not boiling, pour into a bowl

6. Enjoy!

7. Add a few berries or a dash of cream for extra flavor

Nutrition

- Calories: 410 Fat: 38g

- Carbohydrates: 10g Protein: 6g

18. Rhubarb Bread Pudding

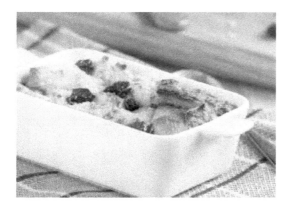

Preparation Time: 15 minutes

Cooking Time: 50 minutes

Servings: 6

Ingredients

- Unsalted butter, for greasing the baking dish

- Unsweetened rice milk – 1 ½ cups

- Eggs – 3

- Granulated sugar – ½ cup

- Cornstarch – 1 tbsp.

- Vanilla bean – 1, split

- White bread – 10 thick pieces, cut into 1-inch chunks

- Chopped fresh rhubarb – 2 cups

Directions

1. Preheat the oven to 350°F.

2. Lightly grease an 8-by-8-inch baking dish with butter. Set aside.

3. In a bowl, whisk together the eggs, rice milk, sugar, and cornstarch.

4. Scrape the vanilla seeds into the milk mixture and whisk to blend.

5. Add the bread to the egg mixture and stir to coat the bread completely.

6. Add the chopped rhubarb and stir to combine.

7. Let the bread and egg mixture soak for 30 minutes.

8. Spoon the mixture into the prepared baking dish, cover with aluminum foil, and bake for 40 minutes.

9. Uncover the bread pudding and bake for 10 minutes more or until the pudding is golden brown and set.

10. Serve warm.

Nutrition

- Calories: 197 kcal Total Fat: 4 g

- Sodium: 159 mg Total Carbs: 3 g

- Protein: 6 g

19. Breakfast Tacos

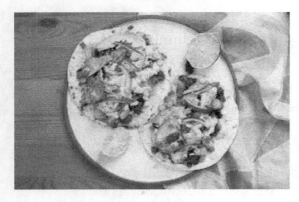

Preparation Time: 10 minutes

Cooking Time: 10 minutes

Servings: 4

Ingredients

- 1 teaspoon olive oil

- ½ sweet onion, chopped

- ½ red bell pepper, chopped

- ½ teaspoon minced garlic

- 4 eggs, beaten

- ½ teaspoon ground cumin

- Pinch red pepper flakes

- 4 tortillas

- ¼ cup tomato salsa

Directions

1. Heat the oil in a large skillet in a medium heat only.

2. Add the onion, bell pepper, and garlic, and sauté until softened, about 5 minutes.

3. Add the eggs, cumin, and red pepper flakes, and scramble the eggs with the vegetables until cooked through and fluffy.

4. Spoon one-fourth of the egg mixture into the center of each tortilla, and top each with 1 tablespoon of salsa.

5. Serve immediately.

Nutrition

- Calories: 331 kcal Total Fat: 11 g

- Sodium: 35 mg Total Carbs: 52 g

- Protein: 6 g

20. Fruit and Cheese Breakfast Wrap

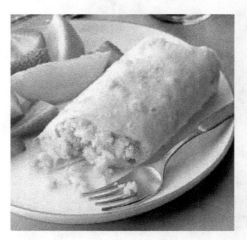

Preparation Time: 10 minutes

Cooking Time: 0 minutes

Servings: 2

Ingredients

- Flour tortillas – 2 (6-inch)

- Plain cream cheese – 2 tbsp.

- Apple – 1, peeled, cored, and sliced thinly

- Honey – 1 tbsp.

Directions

1. Lay both tortillas on a clean work surface and spread 1 tbsp. of cream cheese onto each tortilla, leaving about ½ inch around the edges.

2. Arrange the apple slices on the cream cheese, just off the center of the tortilla on the side closest to you, leaving about 1 ½ inch on each side and 2 inches on the bottom.

3. Drizzle the apples lightly with honey.

4. Fold the left and right edges of the tortillas into the center, laying the edge over the apples.

5. Taking the tortilla edge closest to you, fold it over the fruit and the side pieces.

   Roll the tortilla away from you, creating a snug wrap.

6. Repeat with the second tortilla.

Nutrition

- Calories: 188 kcal

- Total Fat: 6 g

- Sodium: 177 mg

- Total Carbs: 33 g

- Protein: 4 g

21. Hot Breakfast Burrito

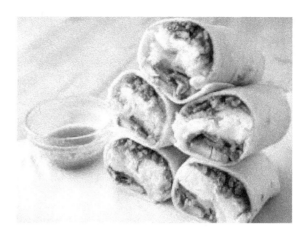

Preparation Time: 5 minutes

Cooking Time: 5 minutes

Servings: 2

Ingredients

- 4 eggs

- 3 tbsp. Ortega green chilies, diced

- 2 flour tortillas, Burrito size

- Nonstick cooking spray

- ¼ tsp. ground cumin

- ½ tsp. hot pepper sauce

Directions

1. Spray a skillet with nonstick cooking spray and heat over medium heat.

2. Beat the eggs with the green chilies, cumin and hot sauce.

3. Pour the eggs into the skillet and cook for 1 to 2 minutes until set.

4. Heat the tortillas for a few seconds in microwave until they are warm.

5. Place half the egg mixture on to each tortilla and roll up burrito style.

Nutrition

- Calories: 366 Total Carbs: 33g

- Net Carbs: 30g Protein: 22g

- Potassium: 245mg

- Phosphorous: 300mg

22. Breakfast Bagel

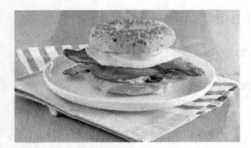

Preparation Time: 5 minutes

Cooking Time: 2 minutes

Servings: 2

Ingredients

- 1 2oz bagel, sliced

- 2 tbsp. cream cheese

- 2 tomato slices

- 2 red onion slices

- 1 tsp. low-sodium lemon pepper seasoning

Directions

1. Toast bagel until golden brown. Spread with cream cheese.

2. Place onion and tomato slice on top.

3. Sprinkle with seasoning.

Nutrition

- Calories: 134 Total Carbs: 19g

- Net Carbs: 17g Protein: 5g

- Potassium: 162mg

- Phosphorous: 50mg

23. Baked Sausage Breakfast Frittata

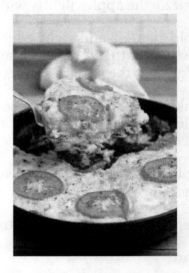

Preparation Time: 15 minutes

Cooking Time: 1 hour

Servings: 9

Ingredients

- 8oz reduced-fat pork sausage, crumbled

- 1 cup cream cheese

- 1 cup 1% low-fat milk

- 4 slices white bread, cubed or broken

- 5 large eggs

- ½ tsp. dry mustard

- ½ tsp. dried onion flakes

Directions

1. Preheat oven to 325 F°.

2. Grease a 9 by 9-inch casserole dish.

3. Cook sausage in a skillet and set aside.

4. Mix cream cheese, eggs and milk in a blender.

5. Stir sausage into the egg mixture.

6. Place bread pieces in prepared dish and pour sausage egg mixture over bread.

7. Bake for 55 minutes or until golden and set.

8. Cut into 9 portions and serve.

Nutrition

- Calories: 223

- Total Carbs: 12g

- Net Carbs: 12g

- Protein: 10g

- Potassium: 208mg

- Phosphorous: 147mg

24. Wheat Berry Breakfast Bowl

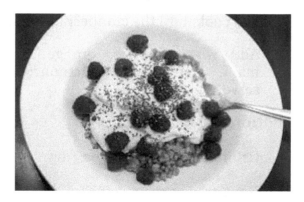

Preparation Time: 20 minutes

Cooking Time: 20 minutes

Servings: 4

Ingredients

- ½ cup wheat berries, uncooked

- 1 medium fresh pear, thinly sliced

- 1 tbsp. butter

- ½ cup fresh cranberries

- 1 tsp. fresh orange zest

- 2 tbsp. maple syrup

- ½ tsp. cinnamon

- 2 tbsp. crystallized ginger

Directions

1. Cook the wheat berries in 1½ cups of water. Bring to the boil and simmer for 30 minutes.

2. Test the wheat berries and cook until al dente for around another 20 minutes.

3. Sauté the pears in the butter until soft. Add the cranberries and ginger and cook until the cranberries burst.

4. Add wheat berries, orange zest, maple syrup, and cinnamon and serve.

Nutrition

- Calories: 174 Total Carbs: 36g

- Net Carbs: 31g Protein: 3g

- Potassium: 220g

- Phosphorous: 90mg

25. Breakfast Pizza

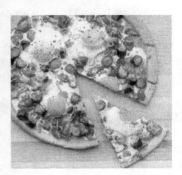

Preparation Time: 10 minutes

Cooking Time: 15 minutes

Servings: 2

Ingredients

- 6 strawberries, sliced

- 1 whole-wheat English muffin

- 1 tbsp. creamy natural peanut butter, unsalted

- 2 tsp. jam, all-fruit

Directions

1. Toast muffin. Spread the muffin with jam and peanut butter. Top with the strawberries and serve.

Nutrition

- Calories: 290 Total Carbs: 45g

- Net Carbs: 38g Protein: 10g

- Potassium: 350g

- Phosphorous: 260mg

26. Asparagus Cauliflower Tortilla

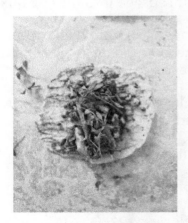

Preparation Time: 15 minutes

Cooking Time: 15 minutes

Servings: 4

Ingredients

- 2 cup asparagus, chopped into bite-size pieces

- 2 cup cauliflower, chopped into bite-size pieces

- 1½ cup onion, finely chopped

- 1 cup liquid low cholesterol egg substitute

- 2 tbsp. fresh parsley, finely chopped

- 2 tsp. olive oil

- Salt and freshly ground pepper

- ¼ tsp. dried thyme

- ¼ tsp. ground nutmeg

- 1 garlic clove, minced

Directions

1. Place the asparagus and cauliflower in a dish with 1 tablespoon of water. Cover the dish and cook on HIGH for around 3 to 5 minutes until tender but also crisp.

2. Sauté the onion in a skillet until translucent.

3. Stir in the vegetables, and remaining ingredients, and reduce the heat.

4. Cook for around 10 to 15 minutes or until set and brown around the edges.

5. Use a spatula to slide the tortilla onto a warm platter or serving plate.

6. Slice into wedges and serve. Also, delicious cold or reheated.

Nutrition

- Calories: 102 Total Carbs: 9g

- Net Carbs: 5g Protein: 9g

- Potassium: 472mg

- Phosphorous: 97mg

27. Baked French Toast Custard

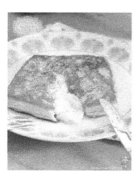

Preparation Time: 15 minutes

Cooking Time: 15 minutes

Servings: 4

Ingredients

- 4 slices of Italian bread. Sliced 1/2" thick

- 4 cup rice milk, non-enriched

- 2 cup liquid low-cholesterol egg substitute

- 4 tbsp. unsalted margarine, melted

- ½ cup sugar

- 1 tsp. almond extract

- 1 tsp. cinnamon

- 1 tsp. powdered sugar or non-calorie sweetener

- Nonstick cooking spray

Directions

1. Spray a 9 by 13-inch baking pan with nonstick cooking spray.

2. Put the bread slices in the baking pan.

3. Beat all the remaining ingredients together.

4. Pour the custard over the bread.

5. Cover the pan and refrigerate overnight.

6. Uncover and bake for 40-50 minutes in a preheated 350 F° oven.

7. Serve warm dredged with powdered sugar.

Nutrition

- Calories: 450 Total Carbs: 65g

- Net Carbs: 64g Protein: 16g

- Potassium: 221mg

- Phosphorous: 111mg

28. Classic Eggs Benedict

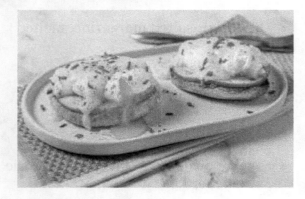

Preparation Time: 15 minutes

Cooking Time: 15 minutes

Servings: 4

Ingredients

- 4oz Canadian bacon, sliced

- 2 English muffins

- 4 eggs & 3 egg yolks

- ½ cup unsalted butter, melted

- 1 tbsp. fresh lemon juice

- 1 dash cayenne pepper

- 1 dash paprika

- 1 tbsp. vinegar

Directions

1. Grill bacon until crisp and keep warm.

2. Slice English muffins in half and toast them.

3. Poach eggs for 3-5 minutes in a large pan of boiling water with vinegar. Keep warm.

4. Beat egg yolks over very light heat.

5. Pour in the melted butter, lemon juice, paprika and cayenne pepper.

6. Beat until thick.

7. Serve with the egg and bacon on top of the English muffins, with a dollop of sauce on top.

Nutrition

- Calories: 416 Total Carbs: 14g

- Net Carbs: 13g

- Protein: 16g

- Potassium: 174mg

- Phosphorous: 214mg

29. Cottage Cheese Pancakes with Fresh Strawberries

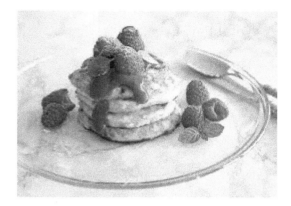

Preparation Time: 20 minutes

Cooking Time: 20 minutes

Servings: 6

Ingredients

- 1 cup cottage cheese

- 4 eggs, lightly beaten

- 6 tbsp. unsalted butter, melted

- 3 cup fresh strawberries, sliced

- ½ cup all-purpose white flour

- Nonstick cooking spray

Directions

1. Mix the cottage cheese, eggs, flour, and melted butter in a large bowl.

2. Spray griddle or frying pan with nonstick cooking spray or butter.

3. Spoon around a ¼ of a cup of batter to form a pancake about 4 inches in size.

4. Cook the pancakes for 2 to 3 minutes on each side.

5. Transfer the pancakes to a heated plate while you cook the rest.

6. Serve the pancakes topped with strawberries.

Nutrition

- Calories: 253

- Total Carbs: 21g

- Net Carbs: 19g

- Protein: 11g

- Potassium: 217mg

- Phosphorous: 159mg

30. Fine Morning Porridge

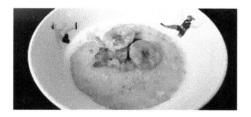

Preparation Time: 15 minutes

Cooking Time: 0 minutes

Servings: 2

Ingredients

- 2 tablespoons coconut flour

- 2 tablespoons vanilla protein powder

- 3 tablespoons Golden Flaxseed meal

- 1 ½ cups almond milk, unsweetened

- Powdered erythritol

Directions

1. Take a bowl and mix in flaxseed meal, protein powder, coconut flour and mix well

2. Add mix to the saucepan (placed over medium heat)

3. Add almond milk and stir, let the mixture thicken Add your desired amount of sweetener and serve

4. Enjoy!

Nutrition

- Calories: 259 kcal

- Total Fat: 13 g

- Total Carbs: 5 g

- Protein: 16 g

CHAPTER 4:

Meat and Poultry Recipes

31. Spiced Pork Roast

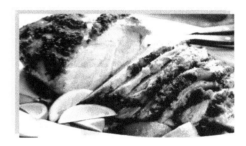

Preparation Time: 10 minutes

Cooking Time: 45 minutes

Servings: 6

Ingredients

- 1 pound boneless pork leg roast

- 2 tablespoons olive oil

- ½ teaspoon black pepper (ground)

- 1½ teaspoons ground cumin

- 1 teaspoon ground cinnamon

- 2 teaspoons chili powder

- 1 teaspoon garlic powder

- 2 teaspoons ground allspice

- Pinch cayenne pepper

Directions

1. In a mixing bowl, add chili powder, allspice, cumin, garlic powder, cinnamon, black pepper, and cayenne pepper. Combine to mix well with each other.

2. Rub pork leg with a spice mix. Refrigerate for 3-4 hours to marinate.

3. Preheat an oven to 350°F. Grease a baking dish with some cooking spray.

4. Take a medium saucepan or skillet, add oil. Heat over medium heat.

5. Add pork leg and stir-cook to sear evenly.

6. Place in a baking dish and bake for about 40 minutes until a thermometer reads 160°F.

7. Slice and serve warm.

Nutrition

- Calories: 117 Fat: 3g

- Phosphorus: 141mg

- Potassium: 252mg

- Sodium: 46mg Carbohydrates: 2g

- Protein: 13g

32. Simple Herbed Pork Chops

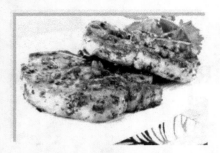

Preparation Time: 10 minutes

Cooking Time: 45 minutes

Servings: 2

Ingredients

- 1 teaspoon black pepper
- ½ teaspoon sage
- ½ teaspoon thyme
- 2 tablespoons vegetable oil
- ¼ cup all-purpose flour
- 4 4-ounce lean pork chops (fat removed)

Directions

1. Preheat an oven to 350°F.Grease a baking pan with some vegetable oil.

2. In a mixing bowl, add flour, thyme, sage, and black pepper. Combine to mix well with each other.

3. Add pork chops and coat well.

4. Place over a baking pan and bake for 40-45 minutes until cooked perfectly and evenly brown.

5. Serve warm.

Nutrition

- Calories: 421 Fat: 23g
- Phosphorus: 204mg
- Potassium: 328mg
- Sodium: 81mg
- Carbohydrates: 13g
- Protein: 19g

33. Steak Burgers/Sandwich

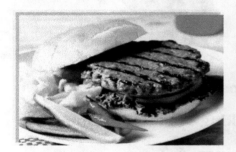

Preparation Time: 10 minutes

Cooking Time: 10 minutes

Servings: 4

Ingredients

- 1 tablespoon lemon juice
- 1 tablespoon Italian seasoning
- 1 teaspoon black pepper
- 4 flank steaks (around 4 oz. each)
- 1 medium red onion, sliced
- 1 tablespoon vegetable oil
- 4 sandwich/burger buns

Directions

1. Season steaks with lemon juice, Italian seasoning, and black pepper. Take a medium saucepan or skillet, add oil. Heat over medium heat. Add steaks and stir-cook for 5-6 minutes until evenly brown. Set aside.

2. Add onion and stir-cook for 2-3 minutes until it becomes translucent and softened.

3. Slice burger buns into half and place 1 steak piece over.

4. Add onion mixture on top. Add another bun piece on top, and serve fresh.

Nutrition

- Calories: 349 Fat: 12g

- Phosphorus: 312mg

- Potassium: 241mg Sodium: 287mg

- Carbohydrates: 9g Protein: 36g

34. Hearty Meatloaf

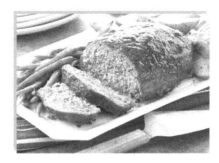

Preparation Time: 10 minutes

Cooking Time: 45 minutes

Servings: 2

Ingredients

- 1 large egg

- 2 tablespoons chopped fresh basil

- 1 teaspoon chopped fresh thyme

- 1 teaspoon chopped fresh parsley

- ¼ teaspoon black pepper (ground)

- 1 pound 95% lean ground beef

- ½ cup bread crumbs

- ½ cup chopped sweet onion

- 1 teaspoon white vinegar

- ¼ teaspoon garlic powder

- 1 tablespoon brown sugar

Directions

1. Preheat an oven to 350°F. Grease a loaf pan (9X5-inch) with some cooking spray. In a mixing bowl, add beef, bread crumbs, onion, egg, basil, thyme, parsley, and black pepper. Combine to mix well with each other.

2. Add the mixture in the pan.

3. Take another mixing bowl; add brown sugar, vinegar, and garlic powder. Combine to mix well with each other.

4. Add brown sugar mixture over the meat mixture.

5. Bake for about 50 minutes until golden brown.

6. Serve warm.

Nutrition

- Calories: 118

- Fat: 3g

- Phosphorus: 127mg

- Potassium: 203mg

- Sodium: 106mg

- Carbohydrates: 8g

- Protein: 12g

35. Hearty Meatballs

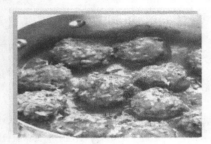

Preparation Time: 10 minutes

Cooking Time: 20 minutes

Servings: 8

Ingredients

Meatball:

- 1 tablespoon lemon juice

- ¼ teaspoon dry mustard

- ¾ teaspoon onion powder

- 1 teaspoon Italian seasoning

- 1 teaspoon poultry seasoning, unsalted

- 1 teaspoon black pepper

- 1 pound lean ground beef or turkey

- ¼ cup onion, finely chopped

- 1 teaspoon granulated sugar

- 1 teaspoon Tabasco sauce

Sauce:

- 1 teaspoon onion powder

- 2 teaspoons vinegar

- 2 teaspoons sugar

- ¼ cup of vegetable oil

- 2 tablespoons all-purpose flour

- 1 teaspoon Tabasco sauce

- 2-3 cups water

Directions

1. Preheat an oven to 425°F. Grease a baking dish with some cooking spray.

2. In a mixing bowl, add all meatball ingredients. Combine to mix well with each other.

3. Prepare meatballs from it and bake in a baking dish for 20 minutes until evenly brown.

4. Take a medium saucepan or skillet, add oil. Heat over medium heat.

5. Add flour, vinegar, sugar, onion powder, mild sauce, and water; stir-cook until sauce thickens.

6. Serve meatballs with sauce on top.

Nutrition

- Calories: 176 Fat: 11g

- Phosphorus: 91mg

- Potassium: 152mg

- Sodium: 61mg Carbohydrates: 6g

- Protein: 14g

36. Beef Pesto Hamburgers

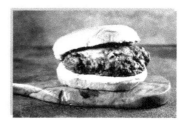

Preparation Time: 10 minutes

Cooking Time: 10 minutes

Servings: 6

Ingredients

- ¼ cup herb pesto

- ½ pound ground beef

- ½ cup chopped sweet onion

- ½ cup shredded cabbage

- 6 hamburger buns, only bottom halves

Directions

1. Take a medium saucepan or skillet; grease it with cooking spray and heat it over medium heat.

2. Add onion and stir-cook until become translucent and softened.

3. Add beef and stir-cook until evenly brown, 2-3 minutes per side.

4. Add cabbage and sauté for 3 minutes.

5. Add pesto, stir mixture, and heat for 1 minute. Arrange buns and add mixture over them.

6. Serve hamburgers fresh.

Nutrition

- Calories: 139 Fat: 2g

- Phosphorus: 124mg

- Potassium: 201mg Sodium: 160mg

- Carbohydrates: 13g Protein: 12g

37. Baked Pork Chops

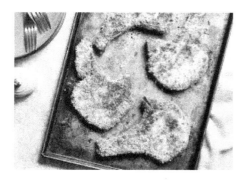

Preparation Time: 05 minutes

Cooking Time: 10 minutes

Servings: 4

Ingredients

- ½ cup all-purpose flour

- 1 large egg

- 1/4 cup water

- 3/4 cup graham crackers crumbs

- 6 center-cut pork chops, 3-1/2 ounces each

- 2 tablespoons unsalted butter

- 1 teaspoon paprika

- 1/8 teaspoon salt

- 6 apple chopped

Directions

1. Preheat oven to 350°F.

2. Combine flour in a flat, shallow pan or plate.

3. Beat egg and water mixture together in a shallow bowl. Place graham crackers crumbs on a shallow plate.

4. Dredge pork chops in flour to coat. Dip each chop in egg mixture then dredge in graham crackers crumbs.

5. Place chops on a baking sheet sprayed with non-stick cooking spray. Drizzle with melted butter.

6. Dust chops with paprika and salt; refrigerate for at least 1 hour.

7. Bake pork chops for 40 minutes or until done.

8. Grill drained apple halves on a grill pan and topped each pork chop with an apple half before serving.

Nutrition

- Calories: 158

- Total Fat: 4.7g

- Cholesterol: 48mg

- Sodium: 86mg

- Total Carbohydrate: 16.8g

- Total Sugars: 8.7g

- Protein: 12.3g

- Calcium: 11mg

- Potassium: 248mg

- Phosphorus: 180mg

38. Balsamic Roasted Pork Loin

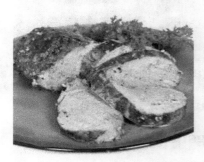

Preparation Time: 5 minutes

Cooking Time: 60 minutes

Servings: 4

Ingredients

- 2 tablespoons basil

- 1/2 cup butter, melted

- 2 pounds boneless pork loin roast

Directions

1. Dissolve basil in balsamic vinegar, then stir in melted butter. Place pork into a resalable plastic bag and pour

marinade over the top. Squeeze out air and seal bag; marinate 2 hours to overnight.

2. Preheat oven to 350 degrees F.

3. Place pork into a glass baking dish along with the marinade. Bake in the preheated oven, occasionally basting until the pork reaches an internal temperature of 145 degrees F, about 1 hour. Let the roast rest for 10 minutes before slicing and serving.

Nutrition

- Calories: 133

- Total Fat: 10.4g

- Saturated Fat: 6.2g

- Cholesterol: 49mg

- Sodium: 85mg

- Total Carbohydrate: 0.1g

- Protein: 9g

- Calcium: 7mg

- Potassium: 156mg

- Phosphorus: 130mg

39. Pineapple Spice Pork Chops

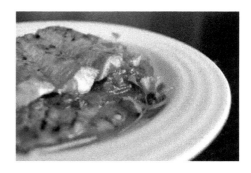

Preparation Time: 10 minutes

Cooking Time: 60 minutes

Servings: 4

Ingredients

- 1 pound pork chops

- 2 tablespoons olive oil

- 1/4 cup honey

- 1/8 teaspoon salt

- 1/4 teaspoon pepper

- 1/4 teaspoon nutmeg

- 1/4 teaspoon cinnamon

- 1 cup pineapples

Directions

1. Preheat oven to broil. Peel and slice pineapples. Broil pork chops in the oven, 4 to 5 minutes on each side.

2. While pork chops are cooking, heat oil in skillet and stir in honey, salt, pepper, nutmeg, cinnamon and pineapples.

3. Cover and cook until pineapples are tender and sauce begins to thicken.

4. Spoon sauce over cooked chops and serve.

Nutrition

- Calories: 255 Sodium: 75mg

- Protein: 12.9g Potassium: 225mg

- Phosphorus: 194mg

40. Pork Meatloaf

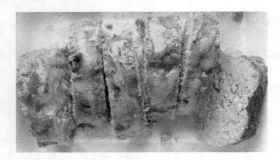

Preparation Time: 10 minutes

Cooking Time: 50 minutes

Servings: 8

Ingredients

- 95% lean ground beef – 1 pound
- Breadcrumbs – ½ cup
- Chopped sweet onion – ½ cup
- Egg – 1
- Chopped fresh basil – 2 Tbsps.
- Chopped fresh thyme – 1 tsp.
- Chopped fresh parsley – 1 tsp.
- Ground black pepper – ¼ tsp.
- Brown sugar – 1 Tbsp.
- White vinegar – 1 tsp.
- Garlic powder – ¼ tsp.

Directions

1. Preheat the oven to 350°F.

2. In a small bowl, stir together the brown sugar, vinegar, and garlic powder.

3. Spread the brown sugar mixture evenly over the meat.

4. Bake the meatloaf for about 50 minutes or until it is cooked through.

5. Let the meatloaf stand for 10 minutes and then pour out any accumulated grease.

Nutrition

- Calories: 103 Fat: 3g
- Carb: 7g Phosphorus: 112mg
- Potassium: 190mg
- Sodium: 87mg Protein: 11g

41. Lemon & Herb Chicken Wraps

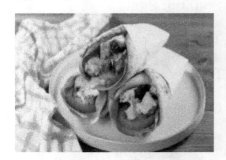

Preparation time: 5 minutes

Cooking time: 30 minutes

Servings: 4

Ingredients

- 4 oz. skinless and sliced chicken breasts
- ½ sliced red bell pepper
- 1 lemon

- 4 large iceberg lettuce leaves

- 1 tbsp. olive oil

- 2 tbsps. Finely chopped fresh cilantro

- ¼ tsp. black pepper

Directions

1. Preheat the oven to 375°F/Gas Mark 5.

2. Mix the oil, juice of ½ lemon, cilantro and black pepper.

3. Marinate the chicken in the oil marinade, cover and leave in the fridge for as long as possible.

4. Wrap the chicken in parchment paper, drizzling over the remaining marinade.

5. Place in the oven in an oven dish for 25-30 minutes or until chicken is thoroughly cooked through and white inside.

6. Divide the sliced bell pepper and layer onto each lettuce leaf.

7. Divide the chicken onto each lettuce leaf and squeeze over the remaining lemon juice to taste.

8. Season with a little extra black pepper if desired.

9. Wrap and enjoy!

Nutrition

- Calories: 200

- Protein: 9 g

- Carbs: 5 g

- Fat: 13 g

- Sodium (Na): 25 mg

- Potassium (K): 125 mg

- Phosphorus: 81mg

42. Sage Pork Chops

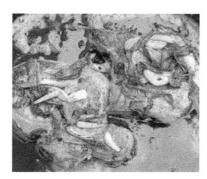

Preparation Time: 10 minutes

Cooking Time: 55 minutes

Servings: 4

Ingredients

- 1 teaspoon dried sage

- 1 teaspoon ground black pepper

- 6 center-cut bone-in pork chops

- 2 tablespoons olive oil

- 1 cup water

Directions

1. Combine the sage and black pepper in a small bowl and rub on both sides of the chops. Heat the olive oil in a large skillet over medium-high heat and sauté the chops for 5 minutes per side, or until well browned.

2. Meanwhile, in a separate small saucepan over high heat. Add water to the chops, reduce heat to low, cover and simmer chops for 45 minutes.

Nutrition

- Calories: 129 Sodium: 33mg

- Protein: 17.6g Calcium: 15mg

- Potassium: 216mg

- Phosphorus: 105mg

43. Beef Tibbs

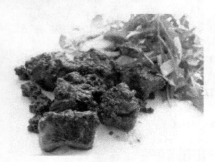

Preparation Time: 10 minutes

Cooking Time: 55 minutes

Servings: 4

Ingredients

- 1 small onion

- 1/2 medium green bell pepper

- 8 ounces lean stewing beef

- 2 tablespoons olive oil

- 1/8 teaspoon salt

- 1/8 teaspoon black pepper

Directions

1. Thinly slice the onion. Chop bell pepper. Cut beef into small cubes.

2. Sauté onion and oil in a skillet until the onion is slightly brown. Add beef.

3. When partially cooked, add bell pepper, salt and pepper.

4. Continue cooking until meat is tender.

Nutrition

- Calories: 181 Sodium: 149mg

- Protein: 18.6g Potassium: 91mg

- Phosphorus: 75mg

-

44. Beef and Macaroni

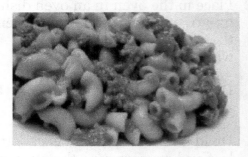

Preparation Time: 15 minutes

Cooking Time: 25 minutes

Servings: 4

Ingredients

- 1 pound ground beef

- 2 cups macaroni

- 1/2 large green bell pepper, coarsely chopped

- 1/2 large onion, chopped

- 2 teaspoons Worcestershire sauce

- 1 teaspoon soy sauce

- 3/4 teaspoon dried basil

- 3/4 teaspoon dried oregano

- 1/2 teaspoon ground black pepper

- 1/2 teaspoon chili powder

- 1/4 teaspoon garlic powder

- 1 cup water

Directions

1. Cook beef in a large skillet over medium heat, occasionally stirring, until browned, about 5 minutes. Transfer beef to a bowl.

2. Cook macaroni, bell pepper, and onion in the same skillet over medium heat for 3 minutes. Add cooked beef, Worcestershire sauce, soy sauce, basil, oregano, ground black pepper, chili powder, and garlic powder. Pour in water. Cover skillet and simmer until macaroni is tender about 15 minutes. Remove lid and simmer, occasionally stirring, until thickened, 5 to 10 minutes.

Nutrition

- Calories: 274

- Sodium: 130mg

- Protein: 29.9g

- Potassium: 456mg

- Phosphorus: 275mg

45. Herbed Pork Chops

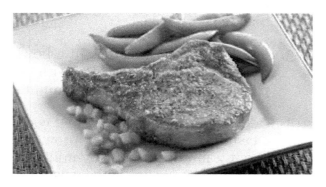

Preparation Time: 10 minutes

Cooking Time: 25 minutes

Servings: 4

Ingredients

- 4 thick-cut pork chops

- 1 teaspoon oregano, or to taste

- 1/2 cup olive oil, divided

- 2 1/2 tablespoons all-purpose flour, or as needed

- 1 tablespoon dried basil

- 1 teaspoon freshly ground black pepper

- 2 cups soy milk

Directions

1. Season pork chops on all sides with oregano.

2. Heat 2 tablespoons olive oil in a large skillet over medium heat. Cook chops into the oil until browned and slightly pink in the center, about 7 to 10 minutes per side. An instant-read thermometer inserted into the center should read at least 145

degrees F. Transfer pork chops to a plate and return skillet to medium-high heat.

3. Mix flour, basil, together in a bowl. Stir black pepper into skillet with the pan drippings and cook for 1 minute.

4. Add flour mixture and cook, constantly stirring, until browned, about 2 minutes. Pour soy milk into flour mixture; cook and constantly stir until mixture is thick and bubbly, 4 to 6 minutes. Pour sauce over pork chops and serve.

Nutrition

- Calories: 349 Sodium: 170mg

- Protein: 9.9g Potassium: 246mg

- Phosphorus: 215mg

46. Lamb with Zucchini & Couscous

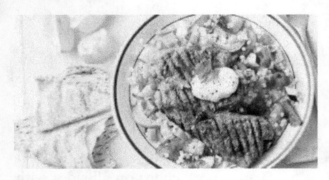

Preparation time: 15

Cooking Time: 8 minutes

Serving: 2

Ingredients

- ¾ cup couscous

- ¾ cup boiling water

- ¼ cup fresh cilantro, chopped

- 1 tbsp. olive oil

- 5-ounces lamb leg steak, cubed into ¾-inch size

- 1 medium zucchini, sliced thinly

- 1 medium red onion, cut into wedges

- 1 teaspoon ground cumin

- 1 teaspoon ground coriander

- ¼ teaspoon red pepper flakes, crushed

- Salt, to taste

- ¼ cup plain Greek yogurt

- 1 garlic herb, minced

Directions

1. In a bowl, add couscous and boiling water and stir to combine,

2. Cover whilst aside approximately 5 minutes.

3. Add cilantro and with a fork, fluff completely.

4. Meanwhile in a substantial skillet, heat oil on high heat.

5. Add lamb and stir fry for about 2-3 minutes.

6. Add zucchini and onion and stir fry for about 2 minutes.

7. Stir in spices and stir fry for about 1 minute

8. Add couscous and stir fry approximately 2 minutes.

9. In a bowl, mix together yogurt and garlic.

10. Divide lamb mixture in serving plates evenly.

11. Serve using the topping of yogurt.

Nutrition

- Calories: 392

- Fat: 5g

- Carbohydrates: 2g

- Fiber: 12g

- Protein: 35g

47. Easy Baby Back Ribs

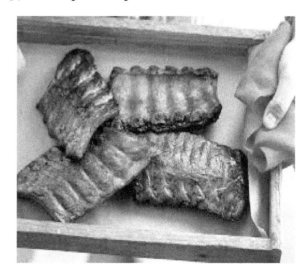

Preparation Time: 05 minutes

Cooking Time: 4 hour 10 minutes

Servings: 4

Ingredients

- 1 teaspoon garlic powder

- 1-1/2 pounds rack baby back ribs

- 3 cups water

- 1-1/2 cups cider vinegar

- 1/4 cup barbecue sauce

Directions

1. Sprinkle ribs evenly (top and bottom) with garlic powder.

2. Coat a top part of broiler pan with cooking spray; place ribs on broiler pan.

3. Pour water and vinegar into the bottom of broiler pan. Put on the top part of the pan with ribs.

4. This allows the ribs to steam.

5. Bake at 300°F for 3-1/2 to 4 hours— don't peek, it lets out steam.

6. Remove foil and brush on barbecue sauce.

7. Cook in the oven an additional 10 minutes.

Nutrition

- Calories: 360

- Sodium: 269mg

- Protein: 18.2g

- Potassium: 86mg

- Phosphorus: 51mg

48. Quick Beef Stir-Fry with Garlic

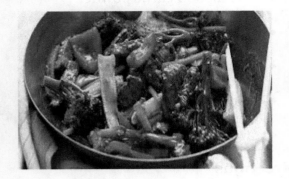

Preparation Time: 10 minutes

Cooking Time: 15 minutes

Servings: 4

Ingredients

- 2 tablespoons olive oil

- 1 pound beef sirloin, cut into 2-inch strips

- 1 1/2 cups fresh broccoli florets

- 1 red bell pepper, cut into matchsticks

- 2 carrots, thinly sliced

- 1 green onion, chopped

- 1 teaspoon minced garlic

- 2 tablespoons soy sauce

Directions

1. Heat olive oil in a large wok or skillet over medium-high heat; cook and stir beef until browned, 3 to 4 minutes. Move beef to the side of the wok and add broccoli, bell pepper, carrots, green onion, and garlic to the center of the wok. Cook and stir vegetables for 2 minutes.

2. Stir beef into vegetables and season with soy sauce. Continue to cook and stir until vegetables are tender about 2 more minutes.

Nutrition

- Calories: 171

- Sodium: 210mg

- Protein: 18.5g

- Potassium: 417mg

- Phosphorus: 200mg

49. Pork with Bell Pepper

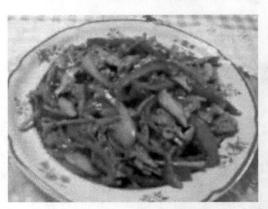

Preparation Time: 15 minutes

Cooking Time: 13 minutes

Serving: 4

Ingredients

- 1 tablespoon fresh ginger, finely chopped

- 4 garlic cloves, finely chopped

- 1 cup fresh cilantro, chopped and divided

- ¼ cup plus 1 tbsp. olive oil, divided

- 1-pound tender pork, trimmed, thinly sliced

- 2 onions, thinly sliced

- 1 green bell pepper, seeded and thinly sliced

- 1 tablespoon fresh lime juice

Directions

1. In a substantial bowl, mix together ginger, garlic, ½ cup of cilantro and ¼ cup of oil.

2. Add pork and coat with mixture generously.

3. Refrigerate to marinate approximately a couple of hours.

4. Heat a big skillet on medium-high heat.

5. Add pork mixture and stir fry for approximately 4-5 minutes.

6. Transfer the pork right into a bowl.

7. In the same skillet, heat remaining oil on medium heat.

8. Add onion and sauté for approximately 3 minutes.

9. Stir in bell pepper and stir fry for about 3 minutes.

10. Stir in pork, lime juice and remaining cilantro and cook for about 2 minutes.

11. Serve hot.

Nutrition

- Calories: 429

- Fat: 19g

- Carbohydrates: 26g

- Fiber: 9g

- Protein: 35g

50. Chicken with Vegetables and Worcestershire Sauce

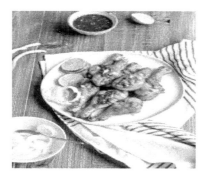

Preparation Time: 15 minutes

Cooking Time: 3 hours

Servings: 2

Ingredients

- 1 cup frozen sliced carrots

- 1 cup frozen green beans

- 1/2 cup diced onion

- 1 pound chicken breasts, boneless and skinless

- 1/2 cup low sodium chicken consommé

- 2 tsp. Worcestershire sauce

- 1 small spoon herb seasoning

Direction

1. Put together carrots, green beans and onion in a pan and cook them slowly.

2. Put the chicken breasts on vegetables and pour the consommé over the chicken.

3. Top with Worcestershire sauce and herb seasoning.

4. Cook at a high heat for 3 hours or low heat for 6 hours.

5. Serve the chicken accompanied by the consommé in a cup and the vegetable mix. Enjoy!

Nutrition

- Calories: 180 Protein: 25 g

- Sodium: 185 mg Potassium: 430 mg

- Phosphorus: 225mg

51. Zesty Turkey

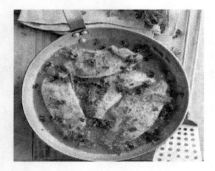

Preparation Time: 15 minutes

Cooking Time: 30 minutes

Servings: 4

Ingredients

- 2 tablespoons balsamic vinegar

- 2 tablespoons butter melted

- 1/4 cup leek

- 1 teaspoon fresh oregano

- 1/2 teaspoon garlic minced

- 1/4 teaspoon black pepper

- 1/4 teaspoon paprika

- 8 ounces skinless, boneless turkey breast

Directions

1. Chop the leek and add to herbs and seasonings. Whisk to combine.

2. Cut turkey into 2 pieces. Pour marinade over turkey in a leak-proof bowl or plastic storage bag. Refrigerate and marinate from 30 minutes up to 24 hours. Remove turkey from marinade. Pan Fry in medium-hot, non-stick or greased skillet for several minutes on each side until thoroughly cooked. (Using a thermometer, the internal temperature of the chicken breast should be 170oF).

Nutrition

- Calories: 258 Sodium: 126mg

- Protein: 25.8g Potassium: 59mg

- Phosphorus: 50mg

52. Sweet and Sour Turkey

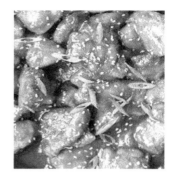

Preparation Time: 15 minutes

Cooking Time: 10 minutes

Servings: 4

Ingredients

- 1 pound boneless, skinless turkey breasts
- 1 cup reduced-sodium chicken broth
- ¼ cup apple cider vinegar
- ¼ cup honey
- 2 teaspoons reduced-sodium soy sauce
- 1/2 teaspoon garlic, chopped
- 1 cup celery, sliced
- 1 small onion, diced
- 1 green pepper, sliced
- 3 tablespoons cornstarch
- 1/4 cup water

Directions

1. Cut turkey into bite-size pieces and place in a saucepan.

2. Add reserved pineapple juice, broth, vinegar, honey, soy sauce and garlic. Cover and simmer over low heat for 15 minutes.

3. Add vegetables and pineapple. Cook 10 minutes, stirring occasionally.

4. Combine cornstarch and water. Gradually stir into the hot mixture. Continue to cook until thickened, stirring constantly.

Nutrition

- Calories: 106 Sodium: 276mg
- Protein: 2.8g Potassium: 212mg
- Phosphorus: 150mg

53. Garlic Chicken

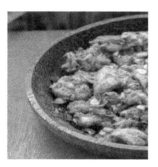

Preparation Time: 10 minutes

Cooking Time: 30 minutes

Servings: 4

Ingredients

- ¼ cup butter
- 2 teaspoons garlic powder
- ¼ cup graham crackers crumbs

- ¼ cup grated Parmesan cheese

- 4 skinless, boneless chicken breast halves

Directions

1. Preheat oven to 425 degrees F.

2. Heat butter and garlic in a small saucepan over low heat until warmed, 1 to 2 minutes. Transfer garlic and butter to a shallow bowl.

3. Bake in the preheated oven until no longer pink and juices run clearly, 30 to 35 minutes. An instant-read thermometer inserted into the center should read at least 165 degrees F.

Nutrition

- Calories: 275 Sodium: 185mg

- Protein: 26.3g

- Potassium: 19mg

- Phosphorus: 15mg

54. Speedy Chicken Stir-Fry

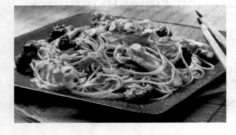

Preparation Time: 10 minutes

Cooking Time: 30 minutes

Servings: 4

Ingredients

- 12 ounces boneless, skinless chicken breast

- 3 tablespoons honey

- 3 tablespoons vinegar

- 3 tablespoons pineapple juice

- 1-1/2 tablespoon reduced-sodium soy sauce

- 1-1/2 teaspoon cornstarch

- 2 tablespoons olive oil

- 3 cups frozen mixed vegetables

Directions

1. Rinse chicken; pat dry. Cut chicken into 1-inch pieces; set aside. Stir-fry frozen vegetables for 3 minutes or until vegetables are crisp-tender. Remove vegetables from skillet.

2. Add chicken to hot skillet. Stir-fry for 3-4 minutes or until chicken is no longer pink. Push chicken away from the center of the skillet. Stir sauce; add to the center of the skillet. Cook and stir until thickened and bubbly.

3. Return cooked vegetables to skillet. Stir all ingredients together to coat. Cook and stir about 1 minute more or until heated through.

Nutrition

- Calories: 197 Protein: 13.4g

- Potassium: 365mg

- Phosphorus: 215mg

55. Super Tender Turkey

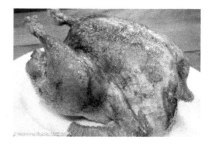

Preparation Time: 10 minutes

Cooking Time: 30 minutes

Servings: 4

Ingredients

- 1 garlic clove
- 1 medium onion
- 1 medium red apple
- 1 tablespoon all-purpose white flour
- 1 -1/2 teaspoons dried rubbed sage
- 1 teaspoon dried thyme leaves
- ½ teaspoon ground allspice
- ½ teaspoon paprika
- 1 pound boneless, skinless turkey breasts
- 2 tablespoons olive oil
- ½ cup apple juice
- 1 tablespoon honey

Directions

1. Mince garlic and thinly slice onion and apples (skin on).

2. Mix flour and all of the spices in a gallon size zip lock bag. Coat turkey breast with the mixture by shaking all ingredients in the locked bag. Heat oil in a large skillet over medium heat. Add chicken and brown on both sides.

3. Remove the turkey from the skillet. Add onions and garlic. Cook and stir 3 minutes or until tender. Add apples. Cook and stir 2 minutes.

4. Stir in apple juice, honey and the cooked turkey, bringing to a boil. Reduce heat to low, cover and simmer 10 to 15 minutes or until desired tenderness.

Nutrition

- Calories: 121 Sodium: 76mg
- Protein: 1.9g Potassium: 162mg
- Phosphorus: 115mg

56. Beef Chorizo

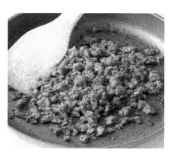

Preparation time: 10 minutes

Cooking time: 10 minutes

Servings: 4

Ingredients

- 3 garlic cloves, minced

- 1 lb. 90% lean ground beef
- 2 tbsp. hot chili powder
- 2 tsp. red or cayenne pepper
- 1 tsp. black pepper
- 1 tsp. ground oregano
- 2 tsp. white vinegar

Directions

1. Mix all ingredients together in a bowl thoroughly then spread the mixture in a baking pan.

2. Bake the meat for 10 minutes at 325 degrees f in an oven.

3. Slice and serve in crumbles.

Nutrition

- Calories: 72
- Protein: 8g
- Carbohydrates: 1g
- Fat: 4g
- Cholesterol: 25mg
- Sodium: 46mg
- Potassium: 174mg
- Phosphorus: 79mg
- Calcium: 14mg
- Fiber: 0.8g

57. Basil Turkey

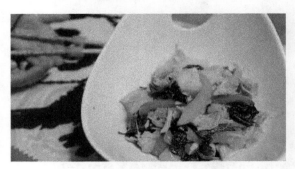

Preparation Time: 10 minutes

Cooking Time: 25 minutes

Servings: 4

Ingredients

- 4 skinless turkey breasts
- 1/3 cup unsalted butter
- 1/4 cup fresh basil
- 1 tablespoon grated Parmesan cheese
- 1/4 teaspoon garlic powder
- 1/4 teaspoon oregano
- 4 fresh basil sprigs

Directions

1. Preheat oven to 325 degrees F.

2. Pierce each breast with a fork several times to allow the mixture to season and flavor as it cooks.

3. Melt butter in a glass mixing bowl in the microwave. Start at 15 seconds and stir to distribute heat.

4. To the melted butter, add basil, Parmesan cheese, garlic powder and

oregano. Stir mixture with a fork or whisk.

5. Pour mixture evenly over turkey breasts making sure parmesan cheese is smoothly distributed.

6. Baked uncovered, basting every 10 minutes with the mixture from the pan, for a total of about 25 minutes or until juices in the chicken are clear, not pink.

Nutrition

- Calories: 209

- Total Fat: 17.9g

- Sodium: 604mg

- Protein: 12.5g

- Potassium: 12mg

- Phosphorus: 10 mg

58. Lamb with Prunes

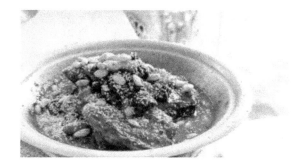

Preparation Time: fifteen minutes

Cooking Time: a couple of hours 40 minutes

Serving: 4

Ingredients

- 3 tablespoons coconut oil

- 2 onions, finely chopped

- 1 (1-inch) piece fresh ginger, minced

- 3 garlic cloves, minced

- ½ teaspoon ground turmeric

- 2 ½ pound lamb shoulder, trimmed and cubed into 3-inch size

- Salt and freshly ground black pepper, to taste

- ½ teaspoon saffron threads, crumbled

- 1 cinnamon stick

- 3 cups water

- 1 cup runes, pitted and halved

Directions

1. In a big pan, melt coconut oil on medium heat.

2. Add onions, ginger, garlic cloves and turmeric and sauté for about 3-5 minutes.

3. Sprinkle the lamb with salt and black pepper evenly.

4. In the pan, add lamb and saffron threads and cook for approximately 4-5 minutes.

5. Add cinnamon stick and water and produce to some boil on high heat.

6. Reduce the temperature to low and simmer, covered for around 1½-120 minutes or till desired doneness of lamb.

7. Stir in prunes and simmer for approximately 20-a half-hour.

8. Remove cinnamon stick and serve hot.

Nutrition

- Calories: 393 Fat: 12g

- Carbohydrates: 10g Fiber: 4g

- Protein: 36g

59. Cabbage Rolls Made with Chicken

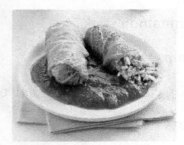

Preparation Time: 15 minutes

Cooking Time: 30 minutes

Servings: 4

Ingredients

- 12 cabbage leaves

- 1 pound ground chicken

- 1/2 cup uncooked white rice

- 1/4 cup onion, finely chopped

- 2 eggs

- 1/2 teaspoon black pepper (divided use)

- 1/4 teaspoon dried basil

- 2 teaspoons dried parsley

- 1-1/4 cup water (divided use)

- 2 tablespoons lemon juice

- 1 tablespoon honey

Directions

1. Carefully remove 12 cabbage leaves from a whole cabbage and wash them. Boil a large pot of water. Add cabbage leaves and cook for 2 minutes to soften. Drain and set leaves aside.

2. In a large bowl, combine ground chicken, rice, onion, eggs, 1/4 teaspoon pepper, basil, parsley and 1/4 cup water.

3. Place 1/4 cup of the chicken mixture on the cabbage leaf and fold sides of the leaf over chicken mixture.

4. Place rolls close together, seam side down in a baking dish.

5. Combine lemon juice, 1 cup water, 1/4 teaspoon pepper and honey to make a sauce. Top cabbage rolls with sauce. Cover and bake at 375 degrees F for 1-1/2 hour. Uncover and bake 30 minutes longer.

Nutrition

- Calories: 243 Sodium: 95mg

- Protein: 25.3g Calcium: 40mg

- Potassium: 292mg

- Phosphorus: 190mg

60. Turkey and Apple Curry

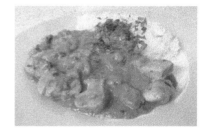

Preparation Time: 15 minutes

Cooking Time: 60 minutes

Servings: 5

Ingredients

- 4 skinless, boneless turkey breasts

- 1/8 teaspoon black pepper

- 1 medium apple, peeled, cored, and finely chopped

- 1 small onion, chopped

- 1 garlic clove, minced

- 1-1/2 tablespoons olive oil

- 1 tablespoon curry powder

- ½ tablespoon dried basil

- 1-1/2 tablespoons all-purpose flour

- ½ cup low-sodium chicken broth

- ½ cup soy milk

Directions

1. Preheat oven to 350 degrees F.

2. Arrange turkey breasts in a single layer in a 9 x 13-inch (or larger) baking dish, adding pepper to taste. Set aside.

3. In a saucepan, sauté apple, onion and garlic in olive oil over medium heat until tender.

4. Add curry powder and basil; mix well, and sauté for another minute.

5. Stir in the flour, and continue to cook one minute longer.

6. Add chicken broth and soy milk, stirring well. Remove from heat.

7. Pour sauce mixture over turkey breasts, and bake for 50 to 60 minutes, or until chicken is done.

Nutrition

- Calories: 238

- Sodium: 67mg

- Potassium: 153mg

- Phosphorus: 140mg

CHAPTER 5:

Seafood and Fish Recipes

61. Grilled Shrimp with Cucumber Lime Salsa

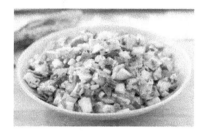

Preparation Time: 15 minutes

Cooking Time: 10 minutes

Servings: 4

Ingredients

- Olive oil – 2 tbsp.

- Large shrimp – 6 ounces, peeled and deveined, tails left on

- Minced garlic – 1 tsp.

- Chopped English cucumber – ½ cup

- Chopped mango – ½ cup

- Zest of 1 lime

- Juice of 1 lime

- Ground black pepper

- Lime wedges for garnish

Directions

1. Soak 4 wooden skewers in water for 30 minutes.

2. Preheat the barbecue to medium heat. In a bowl, toss together the olive oil, shrimp, and garlic.

3. Thread the shrimp onto the skewers, about 4 shrimp per skewer.

4. In a bowl, stir together the mango, cucumber, lime zest, and lime juice, and season the salsa lightly with pepper. Set aside.

5. Grill the shrimp for 10 minutes, turning once or until the shrimp is opaque and cooked through.

6. Season the shrimp lightly with pepper.

7. Serve the shrimp on the cucumber salsa with lime wedges on the side.

Nutrition

- Calories: 120 kcal Total Fat: 8 g

- Cholesterol: 0 mg

- Sodium: 60 mg Total Carbs: 4 g

- Protein: 9 g

62. Shrimp Scampi Linguine

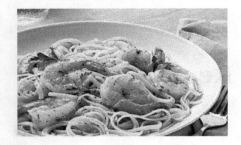

Preparation Time: 15 minutes

Cooking Time: 15 minutes

Servings: 4

Ingredients

- Uncooked linguine – 4 ounces

- Olive oil – 1 tsp.

- Minced garlic – 2 tsp.

- Shrimp – 4 ounces, peeled, deveined, and chopped

- Dry white wine – ½ cup

- Juice of 1 lemon

- Chopped fresh basil – 1 tbsp.

- Heavy whipping cream – ½ cup

- Ground black pepper

Directions

1. Cook the linguine according to package instructions, drain and set aside.

2. Heat the olive oil in a skillet.

3. Sauté the garlic and shrimp for 6 minutes or until the shrimp is opaque and just cooked through.

4. Add the lemon juice, wine, and basil. Cook for 5 minutes.

5. Stir in the cream and simmer for 2 minutes more.

6. Add the linguine to the skillet and toss to coat.

7. Divide the pasta onto 4 plates to serve.

Nutrition

- Calories: 219 kcal Total Fat: 7 g

- Sodium: 42 mg Total Carbs: 21 g

- Protein: 12 g

63. Crab Cakes with Lime Salsa

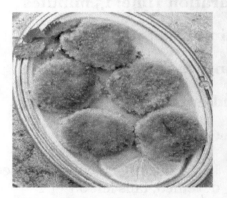

Preparation Time: 20 minutes

Cooking Time: 20 minutes

Servings: 4

Ingredients

- English cucumber – ½, diced

- Lime – 1, chopped

- Boiled and chopped red bell pepper – ½ cup

- Chopped fresh cilantro – 1 tsp.

- Ground black pepper

- For the crab cakes

- Queen crab meat – 8 ounces

- Bread crumbs – ¼ cup

- Small egg – 1

- Boiled and chopped red bell pepper – ¼ cup

- Scallion – 1, both green and white parts, minced

- Chopped fresh parsley – 1 tbsp.

- Splash hot sauce

- Olive oil spray, for the pan

Directions

1. To make the salsa, in a small bowl stir together the lime, cucumber, red pepper and cilantro. Season with pepper and set aside.

2. To make the crab cakes, in a bowl mix the bread crumbs, crab, red pepper, egg, scallion, parsley, and hot sauce until it holds together. Add more bread crumbs, if necessary.

3. Form the crab mixture into 4 patties and place them on a plate.

4. Refrigerate the crab cakes for 1 hour to firm them.

5. Spray a skillet with olive oil spray and place on medium heat.

6. Cook the crab cakes in batches, turning, for about 5 minutes per side or until golden brown.

7. Serve the crab cakes with salsa.

Nutrition

- Calories: 115 kcal

- Total Fat: 2 g

- Sodium: 421 mg

- Total Carbs: 7 g

- Protein: 16 g

64. Seafood Casserole

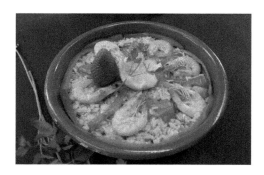

Preparation Time: 20 minutes

Cooking Time: 45 minutes

Servings: 6

Ingredients

- Eggplant – 2 cups, peeled and diced into 1-inch pieces

- Butter, for greasing the baking dish

- Olive oil – 1 tbsp.

- Sweet onion – ½, chopped

- Minced garlic – 1 tsp.

- Celery stalk – 1, chopped

- Red bell pepper – ½, boiled and chopped

- Freshly squeezed lemon juice – 3 tbsp.

- Hot sauce – 1 tsp.

- Creole seasoning mix – ¼ tsp.

- White rice – ½ cup, uncooked

- Egg – 1 large

- Cooked shrimp – 4 ounces

- Queen crab meat – 6 ounces

Directions

1. Preheat the oven to 350°F.

2. Boil the eggplant in a saucepan for 5 minutes. Drain and set aside.

3. Grease a 9-by-13 inch baking dish with butter and set aside.

4. Heat the olive oil in a large skillet over medium heat.

5. Sauté the garlic, onion, celery, and bell pepper for 4 minutes, or until tender.

6. Add the sautéed vegetables to the eggplant, along with the lemon juice, hot sauce, seasoning, rice, and egg.

7. Stir to combine.

8. Fold in the shrimp and crab meat.

9. Spoon the casserole mixture into the casserole dish, patting down the top.

10. Bake for 25 to 30 minutes or until casserole is heated through and rice is tender.

11. Serve warm.

Nutrition

- Calories: 118kcal Total Fat: 4g

- Sodium: 235mg

- Total Carbs: 9g

- Protein: 12g

65. Sweet Glazed Salmon

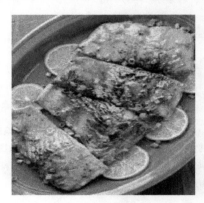

Preparation Time: 10 minutes

Cooking Time: 10 minutes

Servings: 4

Ingredients

- Honey – 2 tbsp.

- Lemon zest – 1 tsp.

- Ground black pepper – ½ tsp.

- Salmon fillets – 4 (3-ounce) each

- Olive oil – 1 tbsp.

- Scallion – ½, white and green parts, chopped

Directions

1. In a bowl, stir together the lemon zest, honey, and pepper.

2. Wash the salmon and pat dry with paper towels.

3. Rub the honey mixture all over each fillet. In a large skillet, heat the olive oil. Add the salmon fillets and cook the salmon for 10 minutes, turning once, or until it is lightly browned and just cooked through.

4. Serve topped with chopped scallion.

Nutrition

- Calories: 240kcal Total Fat: 15g

- Sodium: 51mg Total Carbs: 9g

- Protein: 17g

66. Fish Packets

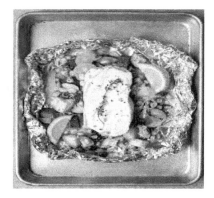

Preparation Time: 15 minutes

Cooking time: 20 minutes

Servings: 3

Ingredients

- 3 tilapia fillets (4 oz. each fish fillet)

- ½ teaspoon cayenne pepper

- ½ teaspoon salt

- 3 teaspoons olive oil

- 1 red onion, sliced

- 3 lemon slices

- 1 zucchini, chopped

Directions

1. Make the medium packets from the foil and brush them with olive oil from inside.

2. Then sprinkle tilapia fillets with salt and cayenne pepper from each side and arrange in the foil packets.

3. Add sliced lemon on the top of the fish.

4. Then add sliced onion and zucchini.

5. Bake the fish packets for 20 minutes at 360F or until vegetables are tender.

Nutrition

- Calories: 161kcal

- Total Fat: 5.9g

- Saturated Fat: 1.8g

- Total Carbs: 6.4g

- Protein: 22.3g

67. Salmon Baked In Foil with Fresh Thyme

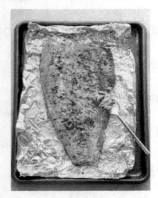

Preparation Time: 10 minutes

Cooking time: 30 minutes

Servings: 4

Ingredients

- 4 fresh thyme sprigs
- 4 garlic cloves, peeled, roughly chopped
- 16 oz. salmon fillets (4 oz. each fillet)
- ½ teaspoon salt
- ½ teaspoon ground black pepper
- 4 tablespoons cream
- 4 teaspoons butter
- ¼ teaspoon cumin seeds

Directions

1. Line the baking tray with foil.
2. Sprinkle the fish fillets with salt, ground black pepper, cumin seeds, and arrange them in the tray with oil.

3. Add thyme sprig on the top of every fillet.
4. Then add cream, butter, and garlic.
5. Bake the fish for 30 minutes at 345°F.

Nutrition

- Calories: 198kcal
- Total Fat: 11.6g
- Sodium: 0mg
- Total Carbs: 1.8g
- Protein: 22.4g

68. Shrimp Paella

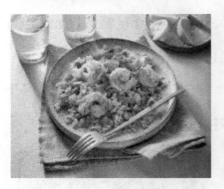

Preparation time: 5 minutes

Cooking time: 10 minutes

Servings: 2

Ingredients

- 1 cup cooked brown rice
- 1 chopped red onion
- 1 tsp. paprika

- 1 chopped garlic clove

- 1 tbsp. olive oil

- 6 oz. frozen cooked shrimp

- 1 deseeded and sliced chili pepper

- 1 tbsp. oregano

Directions

1. Heat the olive oil in a large pan on medium-high heat.

2. Add the onion and garlic and sauté for 2-3 minutes until soft.

3. Now add the shrimp and sauté for a further 5 minutes or until hot through.

4. Now add the herbs, spices, chili and rice with 1/2 cup boiling water.

5. Stir until everything is warm and the water has been absorbed.

6. Plate up and serve.

Nutrition

- Calories: 221

- Protein: 17g

- Carbs: 31g

- Fat: 8g

- Sodium (Na): 235mg

- Potassium (K): 176mg

- Phosphorus: 189mg

69. Grilled Salmon

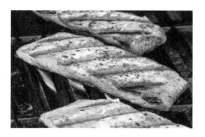

Preparation Time: 15 minutes

Cooking Time: 15 minutes

Servings: 4

Ingredients

- 1 pounds salmon fillets

- 1 tablespoon olive oil

- 1 teaspoon salt-free lemon pepper

- 1/2 teaspoon paprika

Directions

1. Preheat grill on high heat.

2. Spray or brush fillet side of the salmon fillets lightly with oil. Combine seasonings in a small bowl. Sprinkle evenly over fillets.

3. Place salmon directly on the grill, fillet side down. Cook for 4 minutes. Spray or brush skin lightly with oil. Turn fillets over and cook until fish flakes easily with fork, about 3 to 5 minutes.

Nutrition

- Calories: 114 Sodium: 22mg

- Protein: 11.9g Potassium: 80mg

- Phosphorus: 67mg

70. Crab Cakes

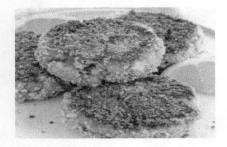

Preparation Time: 15 minutes

Cooking Time: 15 minutes

Servings: 4

Ingredients

- 1 pound crab meat
- 1 egg
- 1/3 cup bell pepper
- 1/4 cup onion
- ½ cup graham crackers
- 1/4 cup reduced-fat mayonnaise
- 1 tablespoon dry mustard
- 1 teaspoon black pepper
- 1 tablespoon fresh parsley
- 2 tablespoons lemon juice
- 1 tablespoon garlic powder
- Dash cayenne pepper
- 3 tablespoons olive oil

Directions

1. Finely chop bell pepper and onion. Crush crackers.

2. Combine all ingredients listed above except the oil; shape into 6 patties.

3. Heat oil in a skillet over medium heat.

4. Cook patties for approximately 4 to 5 minutes, or until browned.

5. Flip patties and cook other side until browned, about 4 minutes.

6. Serve warm.

Nutrition

- Calories: 233 Sodium: 561mg
- Protein: 11.8g Potassium: 83mg
- Phosphorus: 76mg

71. Cod Fish Cakes

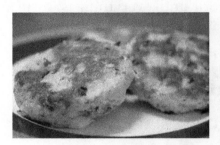

Preparation Time: 15 minutes

Cooking Time: 30 minutes

Servings: 4

Ingredients

- 1 cup broccoli, halved
- 1 pound cod fillets, cubed
- 4 tablespoons olive oil

- 1 tablespoon grated onion

- 1 tablespoon chopped fresh cilantro

- 1 egg

Directions

1. Place the broccoli in a large pot of water, bring the water to a boil. Let the broccoli cook until they are almost tender.

2. Add the fish to the pot and let the fish and broccoli cook until they are both soft. Drain well and transfer the broccoli and fish to a large mixing bowl.

3. Add 1 tablespoon oil, onion, cilantro, and egg to the bowl; mash the mixture together. Mold the mixture into patties.

4. Heat oil in a large skillet over a medium-high heat. Fry the patties on both sides until golden brown. Drain on paper towels before serving.

Nutrition

- Calories: 236 Sodium: 94mg

- Protein: 22.3g Potassium: 92mg

- Phosphorus: 86mg

72. Baked Tuna 'Crab' Cakes

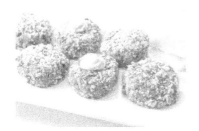

Preparation Time: 20 minutes

Cooking Time: 40 minutes

Servings: 4

Ingredients

- 1 can chunk light tuna in water, drained and flaked

- 1 cup graham cracks crumbs

- 1 zucchini, shredded

- 1/2 green bell pepper, chopped

- 1/2 onion, finely chopped

- 1/2 cup green onions, chopped

- 2 cloves garlic, pressed or minced

- 1 teaspoon finely chopped jalapeno pepper

- 1/2 cup tofu

- 1/4 cup fat free sour cream

- 1 lime, juiced

- 1 tablespoon dried basil

- 1 teaspoon ground black pepper

- 2 eggs

Directions

1. Preheat oven to 350 degrees F. Line a baking sheet with aluminum foil, and spray with cooking spray.

2. Scoop up about ¼ cup of the tuna mixture, and gently form it into a compact patty. And place the cakes onto the prepared baking sheet.

Spray the tops of the cakes with cooking oil spray.

3. Bake in the preheated oven until the tops of the cakes are beginning to brown, about 20 minutes. Flip each cake, spray with cooking spray, and bake until the cakes are cooked through and lightly browned, about 20 more minutes.

Nutrition

- Calories: 63

- Sodium: 74mg

- Protein: 5.3g

- Potassium: 151mg

- Phosphorus: 116mg

73. Lemon Butter Fillet

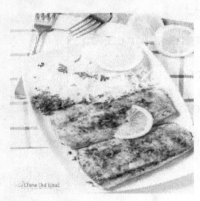

Preparation Time: 20 minutes

Cooking Time: 30 minutes

Servings: 5

Ingredients

- 1/2 cup butter

- 1 lemon, juiced

- 1 teaspoon ground black pepper

- 1/2 teaspoon dried basil

- 3 cloves garlic, minced

- 6 (4 ounce) cod fillets

- 2 tablespoons lemon pepper

Directions

1. Preheat oven to 350 degrees F.

2. Melt the butter in a medium saucepan over medium heat. Bring to a boil.

3. Arrange cod fillets in a single layer on a medium baking sheet. Cover with 1/2 the butter mixture, and sprinkle with lemon pepper. Cover with foil.

4. Bake 15 to 20 minutes in the preheated oven, until fish is easily flaked with a fork. Pour the remaining butter mixture over the fish to serve.

Nutrition

- Calories: 168

- Sodium: 210mg

- Protein: 6.7g

- Potassium: 29mg

- Phosphorus: 16mg

74. Fish Soup

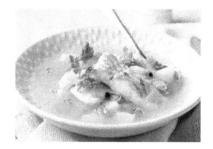

Preparation Time: 10 minutes

Cooking Time: 30 minutes

Servings: 5

Ingredients

- 1/2 onion, chopped
- 1 clove garlic, minced
- 1 tablespoon chili powder
- 1 1/2 cups chicken broth
- 1 teaspoon ground cumin
- 1/2 cup chopped green bell pepper
- 1/2 cup shrimp
- 1/2 pound cod fillets
- 3/4 cup plain yogurt

Directions

1. Spray a large saucepan with the cooking spray over medium high heat. Add the onions and sauté, stirring often, for about 5 minutes. Add the garlic and chili powder and sauté for 2 more minutes.

2. Then add the chicken broth, and cumin, stirring well. Bring to a boil, reduce heat to low, cover and simmer for 20 minutes.

3. Next, add green bell pepper, shrimp and cod. Return to a boil, then reduce heat to low, cover and simmer for another 5 minutes. Gradually stir in the yogurt until heated through.

Nutrition

- Calories: 90 Sodium: 374mg
- Protein: 10g Potassium: 130mg
- Phosphorus: 105mg

75. Baked Fennel & Garlic Sea Bass

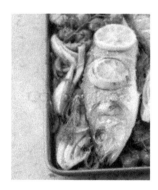

Preparation time: 5 minutes

Cooking time: 15 minutes

Servings: 2

Ingredients

- 1 lemon
- ½ sliced fennel bulb
- 6 oz. sea bass fillets
- 1 tsp. black pepper

- 2 garlic cloves

Directions

1. Preheat the oven to 375°F/Gas Mark 5.

2. Sprinkle black pepper over the Sea Bass.

3. Slice the fennel bulb and garlic cloves.

4. Add 1 salmon fillet and half the fennel and garlic to one sheet of baking paper or tin foil.

5. Squeeze in 1/2 lemon juices.

6. Repeat for the other fillet.

7. Fold and add to the oven for 12-15 minutes or until fish is thoroughly cooked through.

8. Meanwhile, add boiling water to your couscous, cover and allow to steam.

9. Serve with your choice of rice or salad.

Nutrition

- Calories: 221

- Protein: 14g

- Carbs: 3g

- Fat: 2g

- Sodium (Na): 119mg

- Potassium (K): 398mg

- Phosphorus: 149mg

76. Cod Egg Sandwich

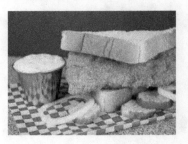

Preparation Time: 10 minutes

Cooking Time: 10 minutes

Servings: 2

Ingredients

- 2 (5 ounce) can cod, drained 6 hard-cooked eggs, peeled and chopped

- 2 cups chopped celery

- 2 tablespoons mayonnaise

- Pepper to taste

- 8 slices white bread

Directions

1. In a medium bowl, stir together the cod, eggs, celery and mayonnaise. Season with pepper to taste. Place half of the mixture onto 1 slice of bread and the other half on another slice of bread.

2. Top with remaining slices of bread. Serve.

Nutrition

- Calories: 181 Sodium: 242mg

- Protein: 14.2g Potassium: 158mg

- Phosphorus: 105mg

77. Tuna Mushroom Casserole

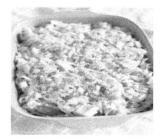

Preparation Time: 10 minutes

Cooking Time: 53 minutes

Servings: 3

Ingredients

- 2 cups macaroni

- 2 (5 ounce) cans tuna, drained

- 1 (10 ounce) can mushrooms, drained

- 1 cup water

- 1 1/3 cups soy milk

- 1/4 teaspoon freshly ground black pepper

- 1 cup dry white bread crumbs

- 3 tablespoons melted butter

- 2 teaspoons dried thyme, crushed

Directions

1. Preheat oven to 350 degrees F. Grease a 1-quart casserole dish.

2. Bring a large pot of water to a boil. Add macaroni and cook for 8 to 10 minutes or until al dente; drain.

3. In a mixing bowl, combine water, milk, and pepper. Mix thoroughly. Then add tuna, mushrooms, and macaroni. Mix thoroughly. Pour mixture into the greased casserole dish.

4. In another mixing bowl, combine bread crumbs, butter, and thyme. Mix well. Sprinkle over the top of the tuna mixture.

5. Bake uncovered in a preheated oven until bubbling and golden brown, about 40 minutes.

Nutrition

- Calories: 264 Sodium: 128mg

- Protein: 15g Potassium: 183mg

- Phosphorus: 85mg

78. Ginger and Lime Salmon

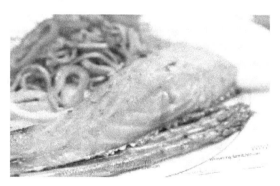

Preparation Time: 15 minutes

Cooking Time: 15 minutes

Servings: 2

Ingredients

- 1 (1 1/2-pound) salmon fillet

- 1 tablespoon olive oil

- 1 teaspoon oregano

- 1 teaspoon ground black pepper

- 1 (1 inch) piece fresh ginger root, peeled and thinly sliced

- 6 cloves garlic, minced

- 1 lime, thinly sliced

Directions

1. Set oven rack about 6 to 8 inches from the heat source and preheat the oven's broiler; if broiler setting has Low setting, set broiler to that. Line a baking sheet with aluminum foil.

2. Season with oregano and black pepper. Arrange ginger slices, salmon and sprinkle with garlic. Place lime slices over ginger-garlic layer.

3. Broil salmon until hot and beginning to turn opaque, about 10 minutes; watch carefully. If broiler has a High setting, turn broiler to that setting and continue broiling until salmon is cooked through and flakes easily with a fork, 5 to 10 more minutes.

Nutrition

- Calories: 59

- Sodium: 10mg

- Protein: 4.5g

- Potassium: 118mg

- Phosphorus: 100mg

79. Lemon Rosemary Salmon with Garlic

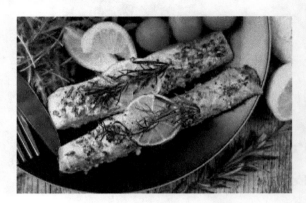

Preparation Time: 15 minutes

Cooking Time: 35 minutes

Servings: 3

Ingredients

- 1/4 cup butter, melted

- 1/4 cup white wine

- 1 lemon, juiced

- 5 cloves garlic, chopped

- 1 bunch fresh rosemary, stems trimmed

- 1 (1 pound) salmon fillet

Directions

1. Preheat oven to 375 degrees F. Mix butter, white wine, lemon juice, and garlic together in a small bowl.

2. Pour a small amount of the butter mixture into an 8x8-inch baking pan until bottom is evenly coated; cover with a thin layer of rosemary. Place salmon, skin side down, into the baking pan. Sprinkle with remaining rosemary; pour remaining butter

mixture over salmon. Cover tightly with aluminum foil.

3. Bake in preheated oven until fish flakes easily with a fork, 25 to 35 minutes. Sprinkle generously with almonds before serving.

Nutrition

- Calories: 103

- Sodium: 62mg

- Protein: 3.1g

- Potassium: 95mg

- Phosphorus: 70mg

80. Lemon-Pepper Salmon with Couscous

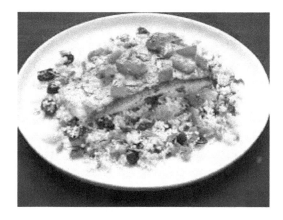

Preparation Time: 10 minutes

Cooking Time: 20 minutes

Servings: 5

Ingredients

- 2 tablespoons olive oil

- 4 (4 ounce) salmon steaks

- 1 teaspoon minced garlic

- 1 tablespoon lemon pepper

- 1/4 cup water

- 1 cup chopped fresh cilantro

- 2 cups boiling water

- 1 cup uncooked couscous

Directions

1. Heat the olive oil in a large skillet over medium heat. Place salmon in the skillet, and season with garlic and lemon pepper. Pour 1/4 cup water around salmon. Place cilantro in the skillet. Cover, and cook 15 minutes, or until fish is easily flaked with a fork.

2. Bring 2 cups water to boil in a pot. Remove from heat, and mix in couscous. Cover, and let sit 5 minutes. Serve the cooked salmon over couscous, and drizzle with sauce from skillet.

Nutrition

- Calories: 134

- Sodium: 27mg

- Protein: 5.7g

- Potassium: 112mg

- Phosphorus: 100mg

81. Sardine Fish Cakes

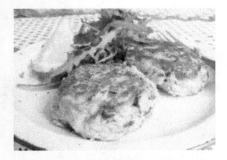

Preparation Time: 10 minutes

Cooking Time: 10 minutes

Servings: 4

Ingredients

- 11 oz. sardines, canned, drained

- 1/3 cup shallot, chopped

- 1 teaspoon chili flakes

- ½ teaspoon salt

- 2 tablespoon wheat flour, whole grain

- 1 egg, beaten

- 1 tablespoon chives, chopped

- 1 teaspoon olive oil

- 1 teaspoon butter

Directions

1. Put the butter in the skillet and melt it.

2. Add shallot and cook it until translucent.

3. After this, transfer the shallot in the mixing bowl.

4. Add sardines, chili flakes, salt, flour, egg, chives, and mix up until smooth with the help of the fork.

5. Make the medium size cakes and place them in the skillet.

6. Add olive oil.

7. Roast the fish cakes for 3 minutes from each side over the medium heat.

8. Dry the cooked fish cakes with the paper towel if needed and transfer in the serving plates.

Nutrition

- Calories: 221 Fat: 12.2

- Fiber: 0.1 Carbs: 5.4 Protein: 21.3

82. Mackerel Skillet with Greens

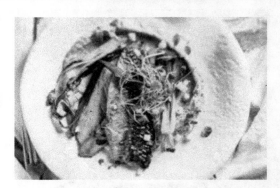

Preparation Time: 10 minutes

Cooking Time: 15 minutes

Servings: 4

Ingredients

- 1 cup fresh spinach, chopped

- ½ cup endive, chopped

- 11 oz. mackerel

- 1 tablespoon olive oil

- 1 teaspoon ground nutmeg

- ½ teaspoon salt

- ½ teaspoon turmeric

- ½ teaspoon chili flakes

- 3 tablespoons sour cream

Directions

1. Pour olive oil in the skillet.

2. Add mackerel and sprinkle it with chili flakes, turmeric, and salt.

3. Roast fish for 2 minutes from each side.

4. Then add chopped endive, fresh spinach, and sour cream.

5. Mix up well and close the lid.

6. Simmer the meal for 10 minutes over the medium-low heat.

Nutrition

- Calories: 260

- Fat: 19.5

- Fiber: 0.5

- Carbs: 1.3

- Protein: 19.2

83. Salmon with Lemon and Dill

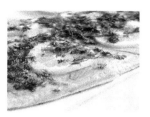

Preparation Time: 10 minutes

Cooking Time: 25 minutes

Servings: 4

Ingredients

- 1 pound salmon fillets

- ¼ cup olive oil

- 5 tablespoons lemon juice

- 1 tablespoon dried dill weed

- ¼ teaspoon garlic powder

- Freshly ground black pepper to taste

Directions

1. Preheat oven to 350 degrees F. Lightly grease a medium baking dish.

2. Place salmon in the baking dish. Mix the oil and lemon juice in a small bowl, and drizzle over the salmon. Season with dill, garlic powder, and pepper. Bake 25 minutes in the preheated oven, or until salmon is easily flaked with a fork.

Nutrition

- Calories: 143 Sodium: 15mg

- Protein: 4.5g Potassium: 133mg

- Phosphorus: 100mg

84. Salmon with Basil

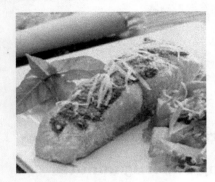

Preparation Time: 10 minutes

Cooking Time: 25 minutes

Servings: 3

Ingredients

- 1 pound salmon fillets or steaks
- ½ teaspoon ground black pepper
- 1 teaspoon onion powder
- 1 teaspoon dried basil
- 2 tablespoons olive oil

Directions

1. Preheat oven to 400 degrees F.

2. Rinse salmon, and arrange in a 9x13 inch baking dish. Sprinkle pepper, onion powder, and basil over the fish. Place pieces of olive oil evenly over the fish.

3. Bake in preheated oven for 20 to 25 minutes. Salmon is done when it flakes easily with a fork.

Nutrition

- Calories: 82
- Sodium: 51mg
- Protein: 4.3g
- Potassium: 93mg
- Phosphorus: 83mg

85. Tuna Casserole

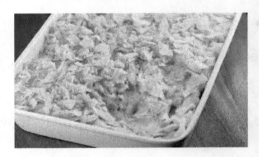

Preparation Time: 15 minutes

Cooking time: 35 minutes

Servings: 4

Ingredients

- ½ cup Cheddar cheese, shredded
- 2 tomatoes, chopped
- 7 oz. tuna filet, chopped
- 1 teaspoon ground coriander
- ½ teaspoon salt
- 1 teaspoon olive oil
- ½ teaspoon dried oregano

Directions

1. Brush the casserole mold with olive oil.

2. Mix up together chopped tuna fillet with dried oregano and ground coriander.

3. Place the fish in the mold and flatten well to get the layer.

4. Then add chopped tomatoes and shredded cheese.

5. Cover the casserole with foil and secure the edges.

6. Bake the meal for 35 minutes at 355F.

Nutrition

- Calories: 260kcal

- Sodium: 0mg

- Fiber: 0.8g

- Protein: 14.6g

86. Curried Fish Cakes

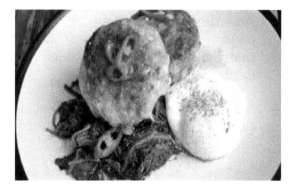

Preparation Time: 10 minutes

Cooking Time: 18 minutes

Servings: 4

Ingredients

- ¾ pound Atlantic cod, cubed

- 1 apple, peeled and cubed

- 1 tablespoon yellow curry paste

- 2 tablespoons cornstarch

- 1 tablespoon peeled grated ginger root

- 1 large egg

- 1 tablespoon freshly squeezed lemon juice

- ⅛ Teaspoon freshly ground black pepper

- ½ cup crushed puffed rice cereal

- 1 tablespoon olive oil

Directions

1. Put the cod, apple, curry, cornstarch, ginger, egg, lemon juice, and pepper in a blender or food processor and process until finely chopped. Avoid over-processing, or the mixture will become mushy.

2. Place the rice cereal on a shallow plate.

3. Form the mixture into 8 patties.

4. Dredge the patties in the rice cereal to coat.

5. Heat the oil in a large skillet over medium heat.

6. Cook patties for 4 to 5 minutes per side, turning once until a meat thermometer registers 160°F.

7. Serve.

8. Increase Protein Tip: To make this a high-protein recipe, use a full pound of cod fillets. The protein content will increase to 28 grams per serving.

Nutrition

- Calories: 188kcal
- Total Fat: 6g
- Saturated Fat: 1g
- Sodium: 150mg
- Total Carbs: 12g
- Fiber: 1g
- Sugar: 5g
- Protein: 21g

87. Shrimp Fettuccine

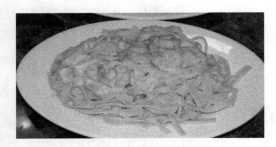

Preparation Time: 20 minutes

Cooking Time: 10 minutes

Servings: 6

Ingredients

- 2 tablespoons olive oil
- 1 leek, white and green parts, chopped
- 12 ounces whole-wheat fettuccine pasta
- 1 cup green beans, cut into 1-inch pieces
- 1 red bell pepper, chopped
- ½ pound medium raw shrimp, peeled and deveined
- 1 cup low-sodium vegetable broth
- ½ teaspoon dried thyme leaves
- 2 tablespoons chopped fresh chives
- 3 tablespoons grated Parmesan cheese

Directions

1. Bring a large pot of water to a boil.
2. Meanwhile, heat the olive oil in a large skillet over medium heat.
3. Sauté the leek for 2 minutes.
4. Add the pasta to the boiling water; cook according to package instructions, until the fettuccine is al dente.
5. Add the green beans and red bell pepper to the skillet and sauté for 2 minutes.
6. Add the shrimp to the skillet and sauté for 1 minute.
7. Drain the pasta, reserving ½ cup cooking water.
8. Add the pasta, broth, and thyme to the skillet and cook for 3 to 4 minutes or until the sauce reduces

slightly and the shrimp curls and turns pink.

9. Sprinkle with the chives and cheese and serve.

10. Increase Protein Tip: To make this a high-protein recipe, use a full pound of shrimp. The protein content will increase to 28 grams per serving.

Nutrition

- Calories: 310kcal

- Total Fat: 60g

- Saturated Fat: 1g

- Sodium: 130mg

- Total Carbs: 48g

- Fiber: 6g Protein: 19g

88. Baked Sole with Caramelized Onion

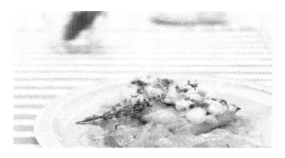

Preparation Time: 10 minutes

Cooking Time: 20 minutes

Servings: 4

Ingredients

- 1 cup finely chopped onion

- ½ cup low-sodium vegetable broth

- 1 yellow summer squash, sliced

- 2 cups frozen broccoli florets

- 4 (3-ounce) fillets of sole

- Pinch salt

- 2 tablespoons olive oil

- Pinch baking soda

- 2 teaspoons avocado oil

- 1 teaspoon dried basil leaves

Directions

1. Preheat the oven to 425°F.

2. In a medium skillet over medium-high heat, add the onions. Cook for 1 minute; then, stirring constantly, cook for another 4 minutes.

3. Remove the onions from the heat.

4. Pour the broth into a baking sheet with a lip and arrange the squash and broccoli on the sheet in a single layer. Top the vegetables with the fish. Sprinkle the fish with the salt and drizzle everything with the olive oil.

5. Bake the fish and the vegetables for 10 minutes.

6. While the fish is baking, return the skillet with the onions to medium-high heat and stir in a pinch of baking soda. Stir in the avocado oil and cook for 5 minutes, stirring frequently, until the onions are dark brown.

7. Transfer the onions to a plate.

8. Remove the baking sheet from the oven and top the fish evenly with the onions. Sprinkle with the basil.

9. Return the fish to the oven and bake 8 to10 minutes longer or until the fish flakes when tested with a fork and the vegetables are tender. Serve the fish on the vegetables.

Ingredient Tip: Frozen fillets can be very high in sodium because they are often frozen in brine. Avoid any frozen fish that provides more than 200 milligrams of sodium per serving. If in doubt, purchase fresh fish.

Nutrition

- Calories: 200kcal

- Total Fat: 11g Saturated Fat: 2g

- Sodium: 320mg

- Total Carbs: 10g Fiber: 3g

- Protein: 16g

89. Veggie Seafood Stir-Fry

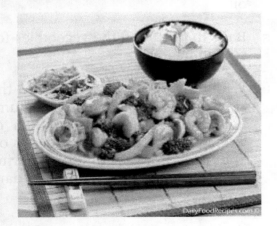

Preparation Time: 12 minutes

Cooking Time: 18 minutes

Servings: 6

Ingredients

- 1 cup low-sodium vegetable or chicken broth

- 1 tablespoon cornstarch

- ½ teaspoon ground ginger

- ⅛ Teaspoon red pepper flakes

- 2 tablespoons olive oil

- 1 onion, chopped

- 2 carrots, peeled and thinly sliced

- 1 pound medium raw shrimp, peeled and deveined

- 1 cup snow peas

- 2 tablespoons sesame oil

- 2 cups cooked brown rice

Directions

1. In a small bowl, combine the broth, cornstarch, ginger, and red pepper flakes and set aside.

2. Heat the oil in a wok or large skillet over medium-high heat.

3. Stir-fry the onion and carrots for 3 to 4 minutes until tender-crisp.

4. Add the shrimp and snow peas and stir-fry for 3 minutes longer or until the shrimp curl and turn pink.

5. Add the sauce and stir-fry for 1 to 2 minutes longer or until the sauce bubbles and thickens. Increase Protein Tip: To make this a high-protein recipe, add 2 cups of frozen, shelled Edam me in step 4. The protein content will increase to 25 grams per serving.

Nutrition

- Calories: 306kcal

- Total Fat: 1.5g

- Saturated Fat: 2g

- Sodium: 127mg

- Total Carbs: 24g

- Sugar: 3g

- Protein: 21g

90. Thai Tuna Wraps

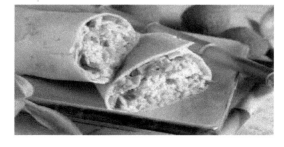

Preparation Time: 10 minutes

Cooking Time: 0 minutes

Servings: 4

Ingredients

- ¼ cup unsalted peanut butter

- 2 tablespoons freshly squeezed lemon juice

- 1 teaspoon low-sodium soy sauce

- ½ teaspoon ground ginger

- ⅛ Teaspoon cayenne pepper

- 1 (6-ounce) can no-salt-added or low-sodium chunk light tuna, drained

- 1 cup shredded red cabbage

- 2 scallions, white and green parts, chopped

- 1 cup grated carrots

- 8 butter lettuce leaves

Directions

1. In a medium bowl, stir together the peanut butter, lemon juice, soy sauce, ginger, and cayenne pepper until well combined.

2. Stir in the tuna, cabbage, scallions, and carrots.

3. Divide the tuna filling evenly between the butter lettuce leaves and serve.

   Ingredient Tip: Make sure to choose light tuna for this recipe, as other types of tuna can contain high amounts of mercury, a dangerous heavy metal. When possible, look for Safe Catch brand tuna because this company only uses fish that is 70 to 90 percent lower than the FDA's mercury limit for albacore tuna.

   Reduce Protein Tip: To make this a low-protein recipe, decrease the tuna to 3 ounces and add 1 cup canned, drained low-sodium chickpeas. The protein content will drop to 13 grams per serving, and the recipe will become high fiber.

Nutrition

- Calories: 172kcal

- Total Fat: 9g

- Saturated Fat: 1g

- Sodium: 98mg

- Total Carbs: 8g

- Fiber: 2g

- Sugar: 4g

- Protein: 17g

CHAPTER 6:

Vegan and Vegetables

91. Cauliflower-Onion Patties

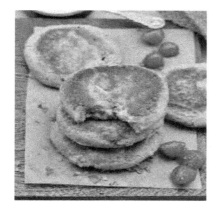

Preparation Time: 5 minutes

Cooking Time: 05 minutes

Servings: 4

Ingredients

- 3 cups cauliflower florets

- 1/2 cup onion

- 2 large eggs

- 2 tablespoons all-purpose white flour

- 2 tablespoons olive oil

Directions

1. Dice cauliflower and chop onion.

2. Boil the diced cauliflower in a small amount of water for 5 minutes; drain.

3. Break eggs into a medium bowl and beat. Add the flour and mix well.

4. Add olive oil to a frying pan and heat.

5. Drop the mixture by spoonful's into the hot oil, making 4 equal portions (or 8 portions is smaller size are desired).

6. Using a spatula, flatten the latkes and fry until brown on both sides.

7. Drain on a paper towel to soak up extra oil.

8. Serve hot.

Nutrition

- Calories: 134

- Sodium: 58mg

- Protein: 5.2g

- Potassium: 286mg

- Phosphorus: 229mg

92. Lentil Vegan Soup

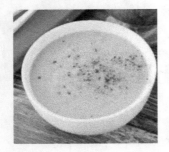

Preparation Time: 10 minutes

Cooking Time: 50 minutes

Servings: 5

Ingredients

- Olive oil – 2 tablespoons

- Onion (diced) – 1

- Garlic (minced) – 2 cloves

- Carrot (diced) – 1

- Potatoes (diced) – 2

- Tomato (diced) – 1 can (15 ounces)

- Dried lentil – 2 cups

- Vegetable broth – 8 cups

- Bay leaf – 1 - Cumin – ½ teaspoon

- Salt – as per taste

- Pepper – as per taste

Directions

1. Start by taking a large pot and add in 2 tablespoons of olive oil. Place the pot over medium flame.

2. Once the oil heats through, toss in the onions and cook for 5 minutes.

3. Add in the garlic and cook for another 2 minutes.

4. Now toss in the diced potatoes and carrots. Sauté for about 3 minutes.

5. Add the remaining ingredients like vegetable broth, tomatoes, lentils, cumin and bay leaf. Once it comes to a boil, reduce the flame to low and cook for about 40 minutes. Remove the bay leaf and season with pepper and salt. Transfer into a serving bowl. Serve hot!

Nutrition

- Fat: 7g Carbohydrates: 58g

- Calories: 364 calories per serving

- Protein: 19g

93. Carrot Casserole

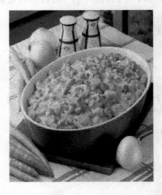

Preparation Time: 15 minutes

Cooking Time: 15 minutes

Servings: 4

Ingredients

- ½ pound carrots

- ½ cup graham crackers

- 1 tablespoon olive oil

- 1 tablespoon onion

- 1/8 teaspoon black pepper

- 1/6 cup shredded cheddar cheese

- Salt

Directions

1. Preheat oven to 350° F.

2. Peel carrots and slice into 1/4-inch rounds. Place carrots in a large saucepan over medium-high heat and boil until soft enough to mash. Drain and reserve 1/3-cup liquid.

3. Mash carrots until they are smooth.

4. Crush graham crackers, heat oil, and mince onion.

5. Place in a greased small casserole dish. Serve hot.

Nutrition

- Calories: 118 Sodium: 86mg

- Protein: 2.4g

- Potassium: 205mg

- Phosphorus: 189mg

94. Chinese Tempeh Stir Fry

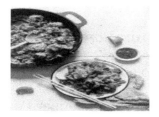

Preparation time: 5 minutes

Cooking time: 15 minutes

Servings: 2

Ingredients

- 2 oz. sliced tempeh

- 1 cup cooked brown rice

- 1 minced garlic clove

- ½ cup green onions

- 1 tsp. minced fresh ginger

- 1 tbsp. coconut oil

- ½ cup corn

Direction:

1. Heat the oil in a skillet or wok on a high heat and add the garlic and ginger.

2. Sauté for 1 minute.

3. Now add the tempeh and cook for 5-6 minutes before adding the corn for a further 10 minutes.

4. Now add the green onions and serve over brown rice.

Nutrition

- Calories: 304 Protein: 10g

- Carbs: 35g Fat: 4g

- Sodium (Na): 91mg

- Potassium (K): 121mg

- Phosphorus: 222mg

95. Broccoli with Garlic Butter and Almonds

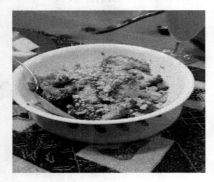

Preparation Time: 10 minutes

Cooking Time: 50 minutes

Servings: 3

Ingredients

- 1 pound fresh broccoli, cut into bite size pieces

- ¼ cup olive oil

- ½ tablespoon honey

- 1-1/2 tablespoons soy sauce

- ¼ teaspoon ground black pepper

- 2 cloves garlic, minced

- ¼ cup chopped almonds

Directions

1. Place the broccoli into a large pot with about 1 inch of water in the bottom. Drain, and arrange broccoli on a serving platter.

2. While the broccoli is cooking, heat the oil in a small skillet over medium heat. Mix in the honey, soy sauce, pepper and garlic. Bring to a boil, then remove from the heat. Mix in

the almonds, and pour the sauce over the broccoli. Serve immediately.

Nutrition

- Calories: 177

- Sodium: 234mg

- Protein: 2.9g

- Potassium: 13mg

- Phosphorus: 67mg

96. Eggplant French Fries

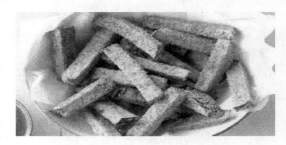

Preparation Time: 10 minutes

Cooking Time: 50 minutes

Servings: 4

Ingredients

- 1 medium eggplant

- 1 cup soy milk

- 2 large eggs

- ¼ cup cornstarch

- ¼ cup dry unseasoned bread crumbs

- ½ cup olive oil

- ½ tablespoon pepper

Directions

1. Peel and slice eggplant into 3/4-inch sticks, 4-inch long. Rinse and pat dry.

2. In a medium bowl, mix milk and eggs until well blended.

3. Heat oil in frying pan on high heat.

4. Place in oil, flipping regularly and fry 3 minutes or until golden brown.

5. Drain on paper towels and serve immediately.

Nutrition

- Calories: 269 Sodium: 112mg

- Protein: 5.5g Potassium: 270mg

- Phosphorus: 167 mg

97. Thai Tofu Broth

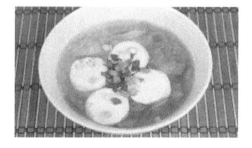

Preparation time: 5 minutes

Cooking time: 15 minutes

Servings: 4

Ingredients

- 1 cup rice noodles

- ½ sliced onion

- 6 oz. drained, pressed and cubed tofu

- ¼ cup sliced scallions

- ½ cup water

- ½ cup canned water chestnuts

- ½ cup rice milk

- 1 tbsp. lime juice

- 1 tbsp. coconut oil

- ½ finely sliced chili

- 1 cup snow peas

Directions

1. Heat the oil in a wok on a high heat and then sauté the tofu until brown on each side.

2. Add the onion and sauté for 2-3 minutes. Add the rice milk and water to the wok until bubbling.

3. Lower to medium heat and add the noodles, chili and water chestnuts.

4. Allow to simmer for 10-15 minutes and then add the sugar snap peas for 5 minutes. Serve with a sprinkle of scallions.

Nutrition

- Calories: 304 Protein: 9g

- Carbs: 38g Fat: 13g

- Sodium (Na): 36mg

- Potassium (K): 114mg

- Phosphorus: 101mg

98. Broccoli Steaks

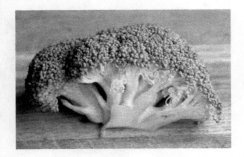

Preparation Time: 10 minutes

Cooking Time: 25 minutes

Servings: 2

Ingredients

- 1 medium head broccoli
- 3 tablespoons unsalted butter
- ¼ teaspoon garlic powder
- ¼ teaspoon onion powder
- 1/8 teaspoon salt
- ¼ teaspoon pepper

Directions

1. Preheat the oven to 400 degrees F. Please parchment paper on a roasting pan.

2. Trim the leaves off the broccoli and cut off the bottom of the stem. Cut the broccoli head in half. Cut each half into 1 to 3/4-inch slices, leaving the core in place. Cut off the smaller ends of the broccoli and save for another recipe. There should be 4 broccoli steaks.

3. Mix butter, garlic powder, onion powder, salt and pepper.

4. Lay the broccoli on the parchment lined baking sheet. Using half of the butter mixture, brush onto the steaks. Place in the preheated oven for 20 minutes. Remove from the oven and flip the steaks over. Brush steaks with remaining butter and roast for about 20 more minutes, until they are golden brown on the edges.

Nutrition

- Calories: 86 Sodium: 143mg
- Protein: 0.8g Potassium: 80mg
- Phosphorus: 61mg

99. Roasted Garlic Lemon Cauliflower

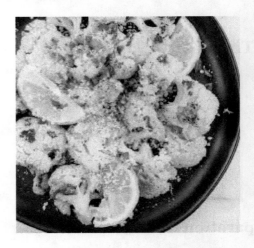

Preparation Time: 10 minutes

Cooking Time: 15 minutes

Servings: 4

Ingredients

- 2 heads cauliflower, separated into florets

- 2 teaspoons olive oil

- ½ teaspoon ground black pepper

- 1 clove garlic, minced

- ½ teaspoon lemon juice

Directions

1. Preheat the oven to 400 degrees F.

2. Bake in the preheated oven until florets are tender enough to pierce the stems with a fork, 15 to 20 minutes. Remove and transfer to a serving platter.

Nutrition

- Calories: 37 Sodium: 27mg

- Protein: 1.8g Potassium: 272mg

- Phosphorus: 161mg

100. Broccoli with Garlic Sauce

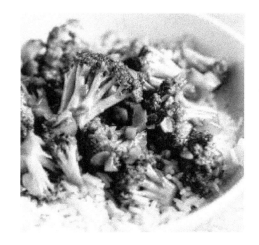

Preparation Time: 10 minutes

Cooking Time: 15 minutes

Servings: 3

Ingredients

- 2 cups broccoli florets

- 1 garlic cloves

- ½ tablespoon butter

- 2 teaspoons honey

- 1-1/2 tablespoons apple cider vinegar

- 1 tablespoon fresh parsley

Directions

1. In a large saucepan with steamer rack, steam broccoli over boiling water 8 to 10 minutes or until crisp-tender (cover with lid while steaming).

2. Stir in honey, apple cider vinegar and chopped parsley. Return saucepan to heat until sauce is heated.

3. Transfer steamed broccoli to a serving dish.

4. Pour sauce over hot broccoli and toss to coat.

Nutrition

- Calories: 41

- Sodium: 26mg

- Protein: 1.4g

- Potassium: 157mg

- Phosphorus: 100 mg

101. Parsley Root Veg Stew

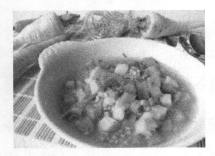

Preparation time: 5 minutes

Cooking time: 35-40 minutes

Servings: 4

Ingredients

- 2 garlic cloves
- 2 cups white rice
- 1 tsp. ground cumin
- 1 diced onion
- 2 cups water
- 4 peeled and diced turnips
- 1 tsp. cayenne pepper
- ¼ cup chopped fresh parsley
- ½ tsp. ground cinnamon
- 2 tbsps. Olive oil
- 1 tsp. ground ginger
- 2 peeled and diced carrots

Directions

1. In a large pot, heat the oil on a medium high heat before sautéing the onion for 4-5 minutes until soft.

2. Add the turnips and cook for 10 minutes or until golden brown.

3. Add the garlic, cumin, ginger, cinnamon, and cayenne pepper, cooking for a further 3 minutes.

4. Add the carrots and stock to the pot and then bring to the boil.

5. Turn the heat down to medium heat, cover and simmer for 20 minutes.

6. Meanwhile add the rice to a pot of water and bring to the boil.

7. Turn down to simmer for 15 minutes.

8. Drain and place the lid on for 5 minutes to steam.

9. Garnish the root vegetable stew with parsley to serve alongside the rice.

Nutrition

- Calories: 210
- Protein: 4g
- Carbs: 32g
- Fat: 7g
- Sodium (Na): 67mg
- Potassium (K): 181mg
- Phosphorus: 105mg

102. Sautéed Green Beans

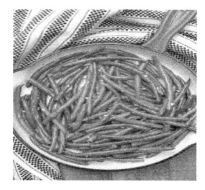

Preparation Time: 10 minutes

Cooking Time: 15 minutes

Servings: 5

Ingredients

- 2 cup frozen green beans
- ½ cup red bell pepper
- 4 tsp. margarine
- ¼ cup onion
- 1 tsp. dried dill weed
- 1 tsp. dried parsley
- ¼ tsp. black pepper

Directions

1. Cook green beans in a large pan of boiling water until tender, then drain.

2. While the beans are cooking, melt the margarine in a skillet and fry the other vegetables.

3. Add the beans to sautéed vegetables.

4. Sprinkle with freshly ground pepper and serve with meat and fish dishes.

Nutrition

- Calories: 67
- Total Carbs: 8g
- Net Carbs: 2g
- Protein: 4g
- Potassium: 192mg
- Phosphorous: 32mg

103. Couscous with Vegetables

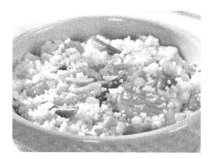

Preparation Time: 10 minutes

Cooking Time: 15 minutes

Servings: 5

Ingredients

- 1 tbsp. margarine
- ½ cup frozen peas
- ½ cup onion, minced
- ¼ cup mushrooms, sliced
- ½ cup couscous, uncooked
- 1 garlic clove, minced
- 2 tbsp. dry white wine

- ½ tsp. dried basil

- ¼ tsp. black pepper

- 1 tbsp. dried parsley

Directions

1. Melt the margarine in a skillet over a medium high heat.

2. Sauté the peas, onion, mushrooms, garlic and wine.

3. Add the herbs.

4. Prepare the couscous according to package Instructions.

5. Toss the vegetables through the hot couscous and serve.

Nutrition

- Calories 104

- Total Carbs: 18g

- Net Carbs: 16g

- Protein: 3g

- Potassium: 100g

- Phosphorous: 52mg

104. Grill Thyme Corn on the Cob

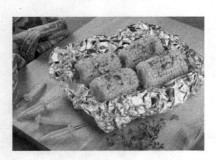

Preparation Time: 10 minutes

Cooking Time: 20 minutes

Servings: 3

Ingredients

- 1 tbsp. grated Parmesan cheese

- 4 half-ear size frozen corn on the cob

- ½ tsp. dried thyme

- ¼ tsp. black pepper

- 2 tbsp. olive oil

Directions

1. In a small bowl, mix the oil, cheese, thyme and black pepper.

2. Coat the corn in the oil mixture.

3. Place the corn in a foil packet topped with 2 ice cubes.

4. Place the corn on a grill and cook for approximately 20 minutes.

Nutrition

- Calories: 125

- Total Carbs: 11g

- Net Carbs: 7g

- Protein: 4g

- Potassium: 164g

- Phosphorous: 57mg

105. Ginger Glazed Carrots

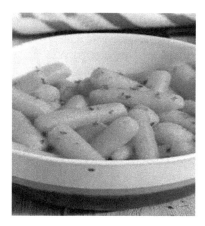

Preparation Time: 10 minutes

Cooking Time: 20 minutes

Servings: 3

Ingredients

- 2 cups carrots, sliced into 1-inch pieces
- ¼ cup apple juice
- 2 tbsp. margarine, melted
- ¼ cup boiling water
- 1 tbsp. sugar
- 1 tsp. cornstarch
- ¼ tsp. salt
- ¼ tsp. ground ginger

Directions

1. Cook carrots until tender.

2. Mix sugar, cornstarch, salt, ginger, apple juice and margarine together 3. Pour mixture over carrots and cook for 10 minutes until thickened.

Nutrition

- Calories: 101
- Total Carbs: 14g
- Net Carbs: 11g
- Protein: 1g
- Potassium: 202g
- Phosphorous: 26mg

106. Carrot-Apple Casserole

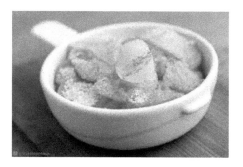

Preparation Time: 20 minutes

Cooking Time: 50 minutes

Servings: 8

Ingredients

- 6 large carrots, peeled and sliced
- 4 large apples, peeled and sliced
- 3 tbsp. butter
- ½ cup apple juice
- 5 tbsp. all-purpose flour
- 2 tbsp. brown sugar
- ½ tsp. ground nutmeg

Directions

1. Preheat oven to 350° F.

2. Boil carrots for 5 minutes or until tender. Drain.

3. Arrange the carrots and apples in a large casserole dish.

4. Mix the flour, brown sugar and nutmeg together in a small bowl.

5. Rub in butter to make a crumb topping.

6. Sprinkle the crumb over the carrots and apples then drizzle with juice.

7. Bake for 50 minutes or until bubbling and golden brown.

Nutrition

- Calories: 106 Total Carbs: 16g

- Net Carbs: 14g Protein: 1g

- Potassium: 206mg

- Phosphorous: 27mg

107. Broccoli-Onion Latkes

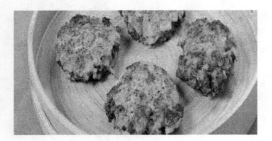

Preparation Time: 20 minutes

Cooking Time: 15 minutes

Servings: 4

Ingredients

- 3 cups broccoli florets, diced

- ½ cup onion, chopped

- 2 large eggs, beaten

- 2 tbsp. all-purpose white flour

- 2 tbsp. olive oil

Directions

1. Cook the broccoli for around 5 minutes until tender. Drain.

2. Mix the flour into the eggs.

3. Combine the onion, broccoli and egg mixture and stir through.

4. Heat olive oil in a skillet on a medium high heat.

5. Drop a ladle of the mixture onto the pan to make 4 latkes.

6. Fry for a few minutes on each side until golden brown.

7. Drain on a paper towel and serve.

Nutrition

- Calories 140

- Total Carbs 7g

- Net Carbs 5g

- Protein 6g

- Potassium 276mg

- Phosphorous 101mg

108. Cranberry Cabbage

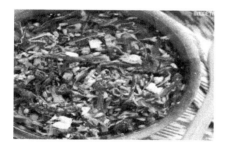

Preparation Time: 10 minutes

Cooking Time: 20 minutes

Servings: 8

Ingredients

- 10 ounces canned whole-berry cranberry sauce
- 1 tablespoon fresh lemon juice
- 1 medium head red cabbage
- 1/4 teaspoon ground cloves

Directions

1. Place the cranberry sauce, lemon juice and cloves in a large pan and bring to the boil.
2. Add the cabbage and reduce to a simmer.
3. Cook until the cabbage is tender, stirring occasionally to make sure the sauce does not stick.
4. Delicious served with beef, lamb, or pork.

Nutrition

- Calories: 73
- Total Carbs: 18g
- Net Carbs: 16g
- Protein: 1g
- Potassium: 138mg
- Phosphorous: 18mg

109. Eggplant Casserole

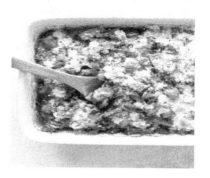

Preparation Time: 15 minutes

Cooking Time: 20 minutes

Servings: 3

Ingredients

- 3 cups eggplant
- 3 large eggs
- 1/8 teaspoon salt
- ½ teaspoon pepper
- ¼ teaspoon sage
- ½ cup white bread crumbs
- 1 tablespoon olive oil

Directions

1. Preheat oven to 350 degrees F.

2. Peel and cut up eggplant. Place eggplant pieces in a pan, cover with water and boil until tender. Drain and mash.

3. Combine beaten eggs, salt, pepper and sage with mashed eggplant. Place in a greased casserole dish.

4. Mix olive oil with white bread crumbs.

5. Top casserole with breadcrumbs and bake 20 minutes or until top begin to brown.

Nutrition

- Calories: 153

- Sodium: 226mg,

- Protein: 7.2g

- Potassium: 221mg

- Phosphorus: 115mg

110. Cauliflower Manchurian

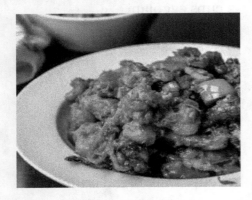

Preparation Time: 15 minutes

Cooking Time: 20 minutes

Servings: 3

Ingredients

- 1 medium head cauliflower

- 1 one-inch ginger root cube

- 1 garlic clove

- 1 teaspoon curry powder

- 1/2 teaspoon chili powder

- 1/2 teaspoon cumin powder

- 2 tablespoons all-purpose flour

- 1 teaspoon lemon juice

- 1 cup olive oil

Directions

1. Separate cauliflower into florets. Finely shred ginger root and mince garlic clove.

2. Combine ginger root, garlic, spices and all-purpose flour. Coat cauliflower uniformly.

3. Heat oil. Drain on paper towels.

4. Drizzle with lemon juice and serve hot.

Nutrition

- Calories: 195

- Sodium: 19mg

- Protein: 1.4g

- Potassium: 186mg,

- Phosphorus: 100mg

CHAPTER 7:

Snacks

111. Parmesan Crisps

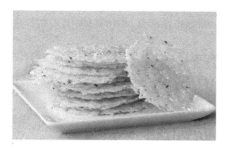

Preparation Time:

Cooking Time:

Servings:

Ingredients

- 2 ounces grated fresh Parmesan cheese (about 1/2 cup)

- 1/4 teaspoon freshly ground black pepper

Directions

1. Preheat oven to 400°.

2. Line a large baking sheet with parchment paper. Spoon cheese by tablespoonful's 2 inches apart on prepared baking sheet. Spread each mound to a 2-inch diameter. Sprinkle mounds with pepper. Bake at 400° for 6 to 8 minutes or until crisp and golden. Cool completely on

baking sheet. Remove from baking sheet using a thin spatula.

Kids Can Help: Let kids sprinkle the grated cheese onto the baking sheets.

Nutrition

- Calories: 31kcal Total Fat: 2g

- Saturated Fat: 1.2g Cholesterol: 6mg

- Sodium: 108mg Protein: 3g

112. Zucchini Dip Ever

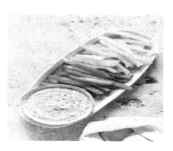

Preparation Time: 15 minutes

Cooking Time: 20 minutes

Servings: 3

Ingredients

- 1 small zucchini, cubed

- ½ tablespoon honey

- 1 tablespoon reduced-sodium soy sauce

- 1 clove garlic, chopped

- ¼ teaspoon dried oregano

- 1 tablespoon low-sodium mayonnaise

Directions

1. Place zucchini in a saucepan, and fill with enough water to cover. Bring to a boil, and cook until tender, about 5 minutes. Drain and transfer to a food processor or blender. Process until smooth. Add the garlic, honey, and oregano and process until blended.

2. Transfer the pureed mixture to a serving bowl and stir in the mayonnaise. Chill for at least 1 hour before serving.

Nutrition

- Calories: 61 Sodium: 510mg

- Protein: 1.4g Potassium: 185mg

- Phosphorus: 60 mg

113. Quick Quiche

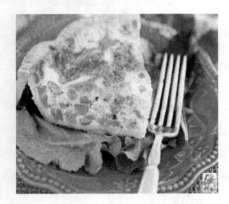

Preparation Time: 15 minutes

Cooking Time: 35 Minutes

Servings: 2

Ingredients

- 1 teaspoon olive oil

- 1 egg white, beaten

- 1 tablespoon finely chopped onion

- ¼ teaspoon black pepper

- ¼ cup all-purpose flour

- ½ cup soy milk

Directions

1. Preheat oven to 350 degrees F. Lightly grease a 9-inch pie pan.

2. Combine egg white, olive oil, onion, black pepper, flour and soy milk; whisk together until smooth; pour into pie pan.

3. Bake in preheated oven for 35 minutes, until set. Serve hot or cold.

Nutrition

- Calories: 121

- Sodium: 48mg

- Total Carbohydrate: 16.5g

- Protein: 5.5g

- Calcium: 21mg

- Potassium: 126mg

- Phosphorus: 90 mg

114. Salmon Sandwich

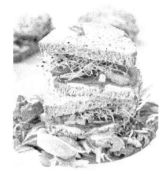

Preparation Time: 10 minutes

Cooking Time: 12 minutes

Servings: 4

Ingredients

- 2 tablespoons olive oil, divided

- 1 tablespoon lime juice

- 1/2 teaspoon lemon-pepper seasoning

- 4 salmon fillets

- 1/4 cup chipotle mayonnaise

- 4 slices sourdough bread

- 1 cup arugula

- 1/2 cup roasted red peppers, diced

Directions

1. Preheat your grill.

2. Coat salmon with half of the oil.

3. Grill salmon for 12 minutes.

4. In a bowl, mix the oil, lime juice and lemon pepper seasoning.

5. Toast the bread in the grill.

6. Spread mayo on the bread and arrange arugula and roasted red peppers.

7. Place salmon on top.

Nutrition

- Calories: 382 Protein: 26g

- Sodium: 384mg Potassium: 640mg

- Phosphorus: 268mg

- Calcium: 45mg Fiber: 1.0g

115. Edamame Guacamole

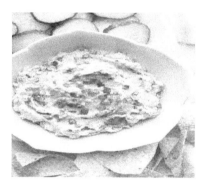

Preparation Time: 10 minutes

Cooking Time: 0 minutes

Servings: 4

Ingredients

- 1 cup frozen shelled edamame, thawed

- ¼ cup water

- Juice and zest of 1 lemon

- 2 tablespoons chopped fresh cilantro

- 1 tablespoon olive oil

- 1 teaspoon minced garlic

Directions

1. In a food processor (or blender), add the edamame, water, lemon juice, lemon zest, cilantro, olive oil, and garlic, and pulse until blended but still a bit chunky.

2. Serve fresh.

   Ingredient tip: Edamame are young soybeans, before they harden, and can be found shelled or in the pods, both fresh and frozen. For convenience, I recommend using the shelled product.

Nutrition

- Calories: 63kcal Total Fat: 5g

- Saturated Fat: 0g Cholesterol: 2mg

- Sodium: 3mg Protein: 3g

116. Chocolate Smoothie

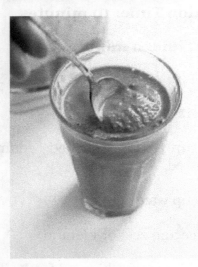

Preparation Time: 5 minutes

Cooking Time: 00 minutes

Servings: 2

Ingredients

- 1 cup pasteurized liquid egg white

- 4 tbsp. whipped topping

- 1 tbsp. chocolate bar shavings

- 1 tbsp. cocoa

- 1 tbsp. cold water

- 1 tbsp. sugar

Directions

1. Mix the cocoa, cold water and sugar together and stir until the sugar has dissolved.

2. Add the egg whites and 3 tablespoons of the whipped topping and stir until the topping is completely combined.

3. Pour into a glass and top with the remaining whipped topping and chocolate shavings.

Nutrition

- Calories: 215

- Total Carbs: 18g

- Net Carbs: 16g

- Protein: 29g

- Potassium: 503mg

- Phosphorous: 78mg

117. Steamed Zucchini

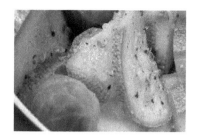

Preparation Time: 05 minutes

Cooking Time: 15 Minutes

Servings: 2

Ingredients

- 2 zucchini
- 2 garlic cloves
- 1 tablespoon olive oil

Directions

1. Bring a large pot of water to a boil. Trim ends from zucchini.

2. Place zucchini and garlic into a steamer basket, then place the steamer basket into the pot. Steam for 10 to 15 minutes, or until the zucchini are tender.

3. Transfer zucchini to a large bowl. Mash the garlic and put it in the bowl with the zucchini. Drizzle the olive oil into the bowl and toss until the vegetables are coated with oil and garlic.

Nutrition

- Calories: 64 Sodium: 20mg
- Total Carbohydrate: 7.1g
- Protein: 2.5g Calcium: 32mg

- Potassium: 520mg
- Potassium: 117mg
- Phosphorus: 101mg

118. Chili Popcorn

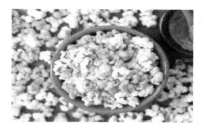

Preparation Time: 10 minutes

Cooking Time: 35 minutes

Servings: 2

Ingredients

- ½ cup unpopped popcorn kernels
- 2 tsp. lime juice
- 1 tsp. chili powder

Directions

1. Prepare popcorn as per package directions. Pour into a large bowl and sprinkle with chili powder.

2. Sprinkle with lime juice and serve.

Nutrition

- Calories: 90 Total Carbs: 18g
- Net Carbs: 15g Protein: 3g
- Potassium: 80mg
- Phosphorous: 70mg

119. Tasty Middle-Eastern Eggplant Dip

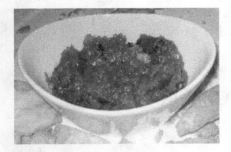

Preparation Time: 10 minutes

Cooking Time: 1 hour 20 minutes

Servings: 8

Ingredients

- 1 head of garlic, unpeeled

- 1 large eggplant, cut in half lengthwise

- 2 tablespoons (30 ml) olive oil

- Lemon juice to taste

Directions

1. With the rack in the middle position, preheat oven to 350°F.

2. Line a baking sheet with parchment paper. Place the eggplant cut side down on the baking sheet.

3. Roast until the flesh is very tender and pulls away easily from the skin, about 1 hour depending on the eggplant's size. Let it cool.

4. Meanwhile, cut the tips off the garlic cloves. Place the cloves in a square of aluminum foil. Roast alongside the eggplant until tender, about 20 minutes. Let cool.

5. Mash the cloves by pressing with a fork.

6. With a spoon, scoop the flesh from the eggplant and place it in the bowl of a food processor. Add the mashed garlic, oil and lemon juice. Process until smooth. Season with pepper.

7. Serve with mini pitas.

Nutrition

- Calories per Serving: 48

- Carbs: 5g Protein: 1g

- Fats: 4g Phosphorus: 17mg

- Potassium: 163mg

- Sodium: 1mg

120. Blueberry Dip

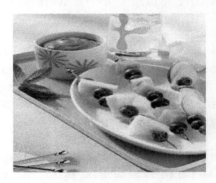

Preparation Time: 10 minutes

Cooking Time: 0 minutes

Servings: 4

Ingredients

- ¼ cup fresh lemon juice

- 1 cup whole fresh blueberries

- 1/3 cup diced red bell pepper
- 2 cups coarsely chopped fresh blue berries
- 2 jalapeno peppers, seeded and minced
- 3 tablespoons chopped fresh cilantro

Directions

1. In a lidded large bowl, mix together bell pepper, jalapeno pepper, cilantro, and lemon juice, whole and chopped blueberries.

2. Cover and refrigerate. You can keep this dip for up to 3 days in your ref and just get a serving each day to bring to work.

3. Also work great as a dip for your Mary's gone crackers.

Nutrition

- Calories per Serving: 71
- Carbs: 18g Protein: 1g
- Fats: 0.5g Phosphorus: 19mg
- Potassium: 138mg Sodium: 2mg

121. Crispy Kale Chips

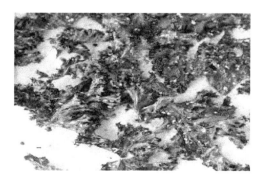

Preparation Time: 10 minutes

Cooking Time: 15 minutes

Servings: 6

Ingredients

- 1 tablespoon olive oil
- 1 teaspoon salt
- 6 cups kale, torn

Directions

1. With cooking spray, lightly grease baking sheet. Preheat oven to 350°F.

2. Remove the kale leaves from its stems and tear into bite sized pieces.

3. Place kale on prepped baking sheet. Drizzle with olive oil and season with salt.

4. Toss kale leaves to coat well with oil and salt.

5. Pop into the oven and bake for 10 to 15 minutes or until leaf edges are turning brown but not burnt.

Nutrition

- Calories per Serving: 28
- Carbs: 2g
- Protein: 1g
- Fats: 3g
- Phosphorus: 15mg
- Potassium: 79mg
- Sodium: 394mg

121. Deviled Eggs

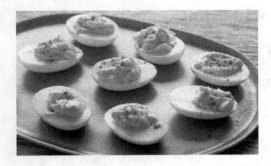

Preparation Time: 10 minutes

Cooking Time: 10 minutes

Servings: 2

Ingredients

- 2 large eggs, hard-boiled and peeled
- 2 tsp. canned pimento
- 2 tbsp. mayonnaise
- ½ tsp. black pepper
- ¼ tsp. paprika
- ½ tsp. dry mustard

Directions

1. Cut the eggs lengthwise in half and remove the yolk.
2. Mix the egg yolk with the dry mustard, mayonnaise and black pepper.
3. Pile the mixture back into the egg whites.
4. Sprinkle with paprika and serve.

Nutrition

- Calories: 90
- Total Carbs: 1g
- Net Carbs: 1g
- Protein: 6g
- Potassium: 94mg
- Phosphorous: 34mg

122. Hot Crab Dip

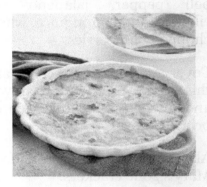

Preparation Time: 10 minutes

Cooking Time: 15 minutes

Servings: 10

Ingredients

- 1 cup cream cheese, softened
- 1 tbsp. onion, finely chopped
- 2 tbsp. 1% low-fat milk
- 6oz canned crab meat
- 1 tsp. lemon juice
- 2 tsp. Worcestershire sauce
- ¼ tsp. black pepper
- ¼ tsp. cayenne pepper

Directions

1. Preheat the oven to 375° F.

2. Mix the cream cheese with the onion, lemon juice, Worcestershire sauce, black pepper and cayenne pepper.

3. Stir in milk.

4. Add the crab meat and stir through.

5. Place mixture into an oven-safe dish.

6. Bake for 15 minutes or until bubbling.

Nutrition

- Calories: 96 Total Carbs: 1g

- Net Carbs: 1g Protein: 5g

- Potassium: 91g Phosphorous: 61mg

123. Greek Turkey Pitas

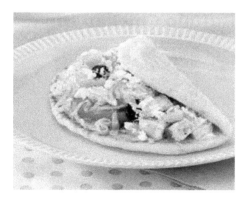

Preparation Time: 10 minutes

Cooking Time: 15 minutes

Servings: 6

Ingredients

- 1½lb ground turkey

- 1 medium onion, chopped

- 1 medium bell pepper, chopped

- ½ cup cucumber, diced

- ½ cup sour cream

- 2 tbsp. olive oil

- 1 ½ tsp. oregano

- 1 tsp. thyme

- ½ tsp. black pepper

- 4 tbsp. red wine vinegar

- 1 large garlic clove

- 6 white pitas, 6-inch size

Directions

1. Brown the turkey in a skillet.

2. Add the onion, garlic, bell pepper, oregano, thyme and black pepper to skillet with turkey and fry until the vegetables are softened.

3. Mix the cucumbers with the sour cream. Toast the pitas.

4. Stuff the pita with the meat mixture and cucumber sour cream.

Nutrition

- Calories: 425 Total Carbs: 37g

- Net Carbs: 34g Protein: 31g

- Potassium: 560g

- Phosphorous: 330mg

124. Apple Bars

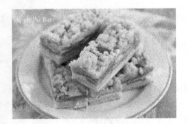

Preparation Time: 20 minutes

Cooking Time: 40 minutes

Servings: 18

Ingredients

- 2 medium apples, peeled and chopped
- ¾ cup unsalted butter
- 1 cup sour cream
- 2 tbsp. milk

What you'll need from the store cupboard:

- 2 cups all-purpose flour
- ½ cup brown sugar
- 1 cup powdered sugar
- 1 cup granulated sugar
- 1 tsp. vanilla extract
- 1 tsp. baking powder
- ½ tsp. salt
- 1 tsp. cinnamon

Directions

1. Preheat the oven to 350° F.

2. Grease a 9 by 13-inch baking pan.

3. Cream the sugar with ½ cup of sugar.

4. Add the apples, sour cream, vanilla, baking soda, salt and flour.

5. Pour the batter into the pan and bake for 35-40 minutes.

6. Make the icing by mixing powdered sugar with remaining melted butter.

7. Drizzle icing over and cut into 18 bars.

Nutrition

- Calories: 247 Total Carbs: 35g
- Net Carbs: 34g Protein: 2g
- Potassium: 71mg
- Phosphorous: 26mg

125. Buffalo Chicken Dip

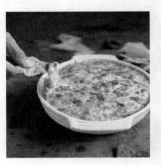

Preparation Time: 10 minutes

Cooking Time: 30 minutes

Servings: 16

Ingredients

- ½ cup cream cheese, softened

- ½ cup bottled roasted red peppers
- 1 cup reduced-fat sour cream
- 2 cup cooked, shredded chicken
- 4 tsp. Tabasco® hot pepper sauce

Directions

1. Puree peppers in a blender.
2. Mix cream cheese and sour cream together in a small bowl.
3. Add pureed peppers and Tabasco sauce.
4. Add the chicken and mix through.
5. Place mixture in a pan and bake in the oven at 350° F for 30 minutes.
6. Serve the dip warm with salad vegetables.

Nutrition

- Calories: 73 Total Carbs: 2g
- Net Carbs: 2g Protein: 5g
- Potassium: 81mg
- Phosphorous: 47mg

126. Chicken Pepper Bacon Wraps

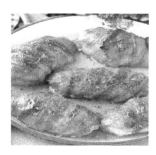

Preparation Time: 20 minutes

Cooking Time: 15 minutes

Servings: 24

Ingredients

- 1 medium onion, quartered
- 12 strips bacon, cut into half
- 12 fresh jalapenos peppers, deseeded
- 12 fresh banana peppers, deseeded
- 2lb boneless, skinless chicken breast, cut into 24 pieces
- 24 toothpicks

Directions

1. Spray grill rack with nonstick cooking spray.
2. Prepare peppers by cutting lengthways on one side of the pepper to split it open.
3. Stuff each pepper with a chicken piece. Place a slice of bacon and onion around each pepper and secure with a toothpick.
4. Grill for around 15 minutes until the bacon is crispy and the chicken is cooked.

Nutrition

- Calories: 73 Total Carbs: 2g
- Net Carbs: 2g Protein: 5g
- Potassium: 81mg
- Phosphorous: 47mg

127. Zesty Duck Wings

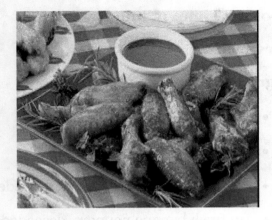

Preparation Time: 10 minutes

Cooking Time: 35 minutes

Servings: 2

Ingredients

- 1 green onion

- ½ tablespoons reduced-sodium soy sauce

- ¼ tablespoon honey

- ¼ teaspoons allspice

- ¼ teaspoons dried thyme

- ½ teaspoon ginger

- ¼ teaspoon minced garlic

- 1/8 cup apple cider vinegar

- 1/8 cup lime juice

- 1/8 cup cranberry juice

- 1 pounds duck wings

Directions

1. Chop green onion.

2. Mix all ingredients except the duck wings. Set aside ¾ cup of marinade.

3. Place duck wings into a container, or large resalable plastic bag. Pour the extra marinade over wings.

4. Cover and marinate in the refrigerator for 4 to 6 hours.

5. Preheat oven to 350°F.

6. Place duck wings on a baking sheet, and bake for 20 minutes.

7. Meanwhile, in a small saucepan, bring reserved 3/4 cup marinade to a boil. Reduce by 1/3 until it thickens slightly to a glaze (approximately 10 minutes).

8. After 20 minutes, remove the duck from the oven and brush wings with the glaze.

9. Raise oven temperature to 400°F and cook duck wings for about another 20 minutes, until done.

Nutrition

- Calories: 78

- Sodium: 23mg

- Protein: 10.4g

- Potassium: 117mg

- Phosphorus: 70mg

128. Yogurt Fruit Dip

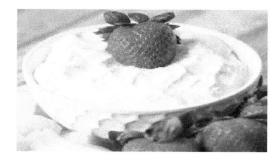

Preparation Time: 10 minutes

Cooking Time: 35 minutes

Servings: 2

Ingredients

- 1 ounce light cream cheese
- 1/4 cup strawberry
- 1 teaspoon cinnamon
- 1 tablespoon honey

Directions

1. Mix ingredients with a hand mixer in a medium mixing bowl until smooth.
2. Refrigerate until ready to serve.

Nutrition

- Calories: 104
- Sodium: 50mg
- Protein: 1.8g
- Potassium: 80mg
- Phosphorus: 40mg

129. Tortilla Wraps

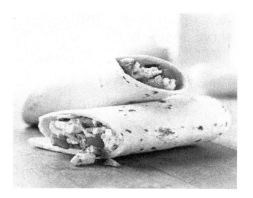

Preparation Time: 5 minutes

Cooking Time: 5 minutes

Servings: 2

Ingredients

- 2 tablespoons carrots
- 2 tablespoons green pepper
- ¼ cup cucumber
- 2 flour tortillas, 6-inch size
- 4 tablespoons whipped cream cheese
- ¼ teaspoon minced garlic
- 1 small onion, chopped
- ¼ cup broccoli

Directions

1. Grate carrots. Chop green pepper and cucumber. Shred chicken.
2. Mix garlic and onion powder into cream cheese.
3. Spread half of the mixture over each tortilla.

4. Add vegetables and meat.

5. Roll up the wrap and refrigerate or serve immediately.

Nutrition

- Calories: 105 Sodium: 179mg

- Protein: 6.5g Potassium: 238mg

- Phosphorus: 196mg

2. Cover with plastic wrap and refrigerate until cold.

Nutrition

- Calories: 63 Sodium: 146mg

- Total Carbohydrate: 4.5g

- Protein: 0.2g Calcium: 3mg

- Iron: 0mg Potassium: 8mg

130. Onion Dip

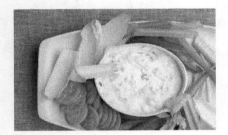

Preparation Time: 10 minutes

Cooking Time: 00 Minutes

Servings: 2

Ingredients

- 1/4 cup mayonnaise

- 1 tablespoon vinegar

- 1 tablespoon Worcestershire sauce

- 1 1/2 teaspoons water, or more as needed

- 1 tablespoon minced onion

Directions

1. Put all ingredients. Add more water as desired for thinner consistency. Stir in minced onion.

131. Popcorn with Sugar and Spice

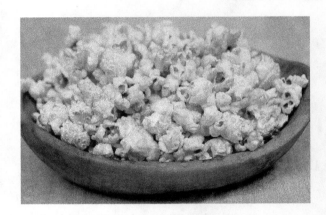

Preparation Time: 5 minutes

Cooking Time: 10 minutes

Servings: 6

Ingredients

- 8 cups hot popcorn

- 2 tablespoons unsalted butter

- 2 tablespoons sugar

- 1/2 teaspoon cinnamon

- 1/4 teaspoon nutmeg

Directions

1. Pop the corn; put aside.

2. Heat the butter, sugar, cinnamon, and nutmeg in the microwave or saucepan over a range fire until the butter is melted and the sugar dissolved.

3. Be careful not to burn the butter.

4. Sprinkle the corn with the spicy butter, mix well.

5. Serve immediately for optimal flavor.

Nutrition

- Calories: 120kcal Sodium: 2mg

- Total Carbs: 12g Protein: 2g

132. Spicy Strawberry Plums Peach Salsa

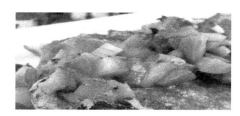

Preparation Time: 20 minutes

Cooking Time: 0 minutes

Servings: 2

Ingredients

- 1 ripe peach – peeled, pitted, and diced

- 2 plums diced

- 2 fresh strawberries, diced

- ¼ jalapeno pepper, seeded and diced

- ½ tablespoon lime juice

- ¼ teaspoon honey

- ½ green onion, chopped

- 1 tablespoon chopped fresh cilantro

Directions

1. Combine the peach, plums, strawberries, jalapeno pepper, lime juice, green onion, cilantro, and honey in a bowl; gently stir to combine.

Nutrition

- Calories: 68 Sodium: 1mg

- Protein: 1.4g Potassium: 194mg

- Phosphorus: 140mg

133. Caraway Seeds and Lemon Biscotti

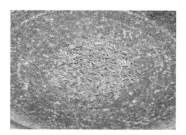

Preparation Time: 15 minutes

Cooking Time: 10 Minutes

Servings: 18

Ingredients

- 2-1/2 cups all-purpose flour

- 2 teaspoons baking powder

- 2 teaspoons caraway seed

- 1 teaspoon grated lemon peel

- ½ cup honey

- 1 large egg white

- 2 tablespoons olive oil

- 1 teaspoon lemon juice

Directions

1. Preheat oven to 350 degrees F. Line a large cookie sheet with parchment paper.

2. Mix first five ingredients (all-purpose flour, baking powder, caraway seed, and lemon peel) in a large bowl and stir well.

3. Place egg white, oil, and lemon juice, honey in a small bowl, and beat until frothy, either by hand with a whisk or with an electric mixer for about 30 seconds.

4. Pour liquid mixture into dry ingredients. Mix with a wooden spoon until dough is mixed. Can use low speed on a mixer for about 1 minute.

5. Place dough on a lightly floured board and shape into a ball. Cut in half.

6. Roll each half into a log approximately 12" long. Flatten top slightly.

7. Remove from oven. Use a bread knife or other serrated knife and slice at approximately 3/4" intervals to get 18 biscotti per half of dough.

8. Place sliced biscotti back on cookie sheet with cut side up and bake until lightly golden, approximately 5 minutes. Remove from oven, turn biscotti over and bake 5 minutes. Remove from oven and cool on a rack.

Nutrition

- Calories: 95 Sodium: 3mg

- Protein: 1.7g Calcium: 29mg

- Potassium: 83mg

- Phosphorus: 76 mg

134. Spicy Broccoli Macaroni

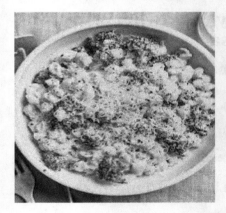

Preparation Time: 10 minutes

Cooking Time: 25 Minutes

Servings: 2

Ingredients

- 1 cup boiled macaroni

- 2 tsp. garlic, chopped

- 1/2 tsp. red chilies, chopped
- ¼ cup broccoli
- Pepper
- Olive oil

Directions

1. Heat oil in a pan and sauté the garlic.
2. Add red chilies. Season with salt and pepper.
3. Add broccoli and cook for two minutes.
4. Add boiled macaroni.
5. Cook for 2-3 minutes. Serve hot.

Nutrition

- Calories: 102 Sodium: 35mg
- Protein: 3.4g Calcium: 39mg
- Potassium: 39mg
- Phosphorus: 10 mg

135. Chicken in Lettuce Wraps

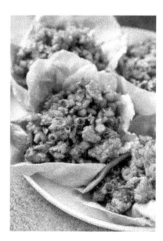

Preparation Time: 20 minutes

Cooking Time: 15 minutes

Servings: 4

Ingredients

- 8 oz. chicken breast, cooked and cubed
- 2 scallions, chopped
- 2 teaspoons garlic, minced
- 2 tablespoons vegetable oil
- 1 tablespoon sesame oil
- 2 tablespoons rice vinegar
- 2 teaspoons hoisin sauce
- 1/4 cup onion,
- 1/4 cup fresh cilantro
- 1/4 cup mushroom
- 8 lettuce leaves

Directions

1. Mix all the ingredients in a pan over medium heat, except the onion, cilantro, mushroom and lettuce.
2. Cook for 15 minutes.
3. Remove the chicken and drain.
4. Place chicken cubes on top of each lettuce leaf.
5. Top with the onion, mushroom and cilantro.
6. Wrap and secure.

Nutrition

- Calories: 219
- Protein: 17g
- Carbohydrates: 4g
- Fat: 15g
- Cholesterol: 51mg
- Sodium: 103mg
- Potassium: 225mg
- Phosphorus: 130mg
- Calcium: 25mg
- Fiber: 0.8g

136. Egg & Salsa Sandwich

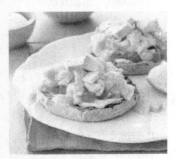

Preparation Time: 5 minutes

Cooking Time: 5 minutes

Servings: 4

Ingredients

- 2 tablespoons olive oil
- 6 eggs, beaten
- 8 slices white bread

- 4 teaspoons salsa

Directions

1. Pour oil in a pan over medium heat.
2. Cook scrambled eggs until firm.
3. Top white bread with salsa and eggs.
4. Place another slice on top.

Nutrition

- Calories: 327 Protein: 16g
- Sodium: 318mg Potassium: 177mg
- Phosphorus: 272mg
- Calcium: 90mg Fiber: 6.0g

137. Apple Cheese Pizza

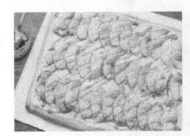

Preparation Time: 10 minutes

Cooking Time: 30 minutes

Servings: 2

Ingredients

- 1/4 cup cream cheese
- 1 (6inch) prepared pizza crust
- 1 large apple
- 1/2 cups shredded goat cheese

Directions

1. Preheat oven to 450 degrees F.

2. Spread cream cheese over pizza crust and arrange apple slices to cover crust. Sprinkle cheese on top. Bake for 30 minutes in preheated oven.

Nutrition

- Calories: 136 Sodium: 173mg

- Protein: 3.6g Potassium: 79mg

- Phosphorus: 40mg

138. Baked Apple Chips

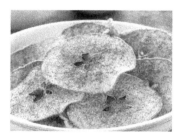

Preparation Time: 10 minutes

Cooking Time: 120 minutes

Servings: 2

Ingredients

- ½ tablespoon honey

- ¼ tablespoon ground allspice

- 1 Granny Smith apples, cored and sliced into very thin rounds

Directions

1. Preheat oven to 250 degrees F. Line two baking sheets with parchment paper.

2. Whisk honey and allspice together in a large bowl. Add apple slices and toss to coat. Arrange apple slices in a single layer on prepared baking sheets.

3. Bake apples in the preheated oven until browned and just crisped about 2 hours. Cool completely.

Nutrition

- Calories: 38 Sodium: 1mg

- Protein: 0.2g Potassium: 63mg

- Phosphorus: 20mg

139. Spicy Pineapple Sauce

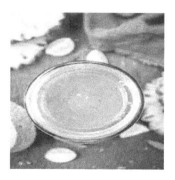

Preparation Time: 20 minutes

Cooking Time: 25 minutes

Servings: 2

Ingredients

- ½ cup crushed pineapple

- ¼ teaspoon ground ginger

- ¼ cup apple juice

- 1 tablespoon honey

Directions

1. In a medium bowl, mix the crushed pineapple, and ground ginger. Gradually stir in enough of the reserved pineapple juice to make the mixture smooth.

2. In a medium saucepan over medium heat, blend apple juice and honey. Cook and stir 5 minutes, until clear and thickened. Mix in the pineapple mixture. Continue to cook and stir until well blended and thick, about 15 minutes.

Nutrition

- Calories: 34 Sodium: 1mg

- Protein: 0.3g Potassium: 58mg

- Phosphorus: 40mg

140. Cauliflower Lovers Dip

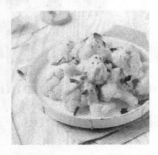

Preparation Time: 10 minutes

Cooking Time: 00 Minutes

Servings: 2

Ingredients

- ¼ cup cream cheese, softened

- ¼ cup cauliflower chopped and cooked

- ¼ tablespoon ketchup

- ¼ cup firm tofu, drained and cubed

- 1 carrot, shredded

- 2 tablespoons Worcestershire sauce

- 1 head lettuce leaves, separated

Directions

1. In a saucepan combine the water and rice. Bring to a boil, cover, and reduce heat to a simmer. Simmer for 20 minutes, until water is absorbed. Set aside and keep warm.

2. Heat oil in a wok over medium-high heat. Cook the pork, green onions, and garlic for 5 to 7 minutes, or until lightly brown. Add the tofu, carrot, and Worcestershire sauce, stirring frequently until heated through. Remove from heat, and stir in the olive oil.

   To serve: spoon a small amount of rice into each lettuce leaf, top with the stir-fry mixture, and drizzle with additional Worcestershire sauce, if desired. Wrap the lettuce leaf to enclose the filling.

Nutrition

- Calories: 108 Sodium: 378mg

- Total Carbohydrate: 18.8g

- Protein: 3.2g Calcium: 43mg

- Iron: 3mg

- Potassium: 188mg

- Phosphorus: 145mg

CHAPTER 8:

Soups and Salads

141. Chicken and Corn Soup

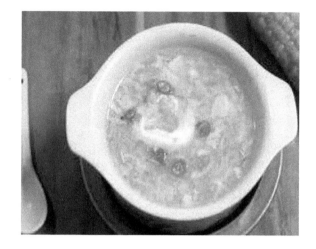

Preparation Time: 30 minutes

Cooking Time 3 hours

Servings: 12

Ingredients

- 4lb roasting chicken

- 3 cup medium-size flat noodles, uncooked

- 2 cans unsalted corn, drained

- 1 tbsp. dried parsley

- ¼ tsp. black pepper

- 14 cup water

Directions

1. Cook the chicken in a large pot with 8 cups of water.

2. Reserve the broth and after cooling the chicken, chop meat into small pieces.

3. Cook noodles according to package Instructions, drain and set aside.

4. Place 6 cups of water, 6 cups of broth, cooked chicken, cooked noodles, corn, parsley and pepper into a large stockpot.

5. Bring to the boil, simmer and serve.

Nutrition

- Calories: 222

- Total Carbs: 17g

- Net Carbs: 15g

- Protein: 25g

- Potassium: 303mg

- Phosphorous: 212mg

142. Creamy Broccoli Soup

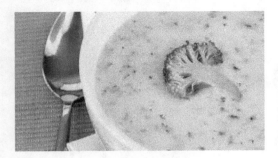

Preparation Time: 10 minutes

Cooking Time: 15 minutes

Servings: 4

Ingredients

- 1 cup broccoli florets

- 1¼ cup kidney beans, cooked

- 2 cup fat-free milk

- 1 tsp. ground oregano

- ½ tsp. garlic powder

- ¼ tsp. ground black pepper

Directions

1. Cook the broccoli in a steamer until tender-crisp for around 7 minutes,

2. Place the broccoli, beans and milk in a blender and puree.

3. Return the soup to the pan add the garlic and oregano and simmer for a further 7 minutes before serving.

Nutrition

- Calories: 130

- Total Carbs: 22g

- Net Carbs: 16g

- Protein: 11g

- Potassium: 650mg

- Phosphorous: 250mg

143. Cabbage Borscht

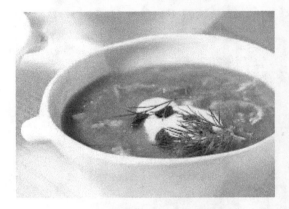

Preparation Time: 30 minutes

Cooking Time: 3 hours

Servings: 12

Ingredients

- 1 medium cabbage, shredded

- 1 cup onion, chopped

- 1 cup carrots, chopped

- 1 cup turnips, chopped

- 2lb beef blade steaks

- 6 cup cold water

- 2 tbsp. olive oil

- ½ cup low-sodium tomato sauce

- ¾ tsp. salt

- 1 tsp. pepper

- 6 tbsp. lemon juice

- 4 tbsp. sugar

Directions

1. Place steak in a stockpot and cover with water. Cover with a lid and boil the meat until it shreds easily.

2. Allow the beef to cool and then shred.

3. Season with salt and pepper and cook for around 1 hour until the vegetables are tender.

Nutrition

- Calories: 202

- Total Carbs: 9g

- Net Carbs: 7g

- Protein: 19g

- Potassium: 388g

- Phosphorous: 160mg

144. Green Pea Salad

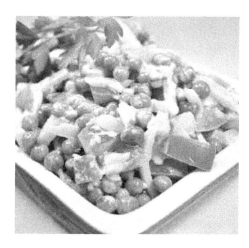

Preparation Time: 10 minutes

Cooking Time: 0 minutes

Servings: 4

Ingredients

- ¼ cup red onion, chopped

- 2 fresh basil leaves, minced

- ¼ cup plain, low-fat Greek yogurt

- 1½ cup frozen green peas

- ¼ cup shredded mozzarella cheese

- 2 tbsp. mayonnaise

Directions

1. In a small bowl, combine the yogurt and mayonnaise.

2. Boil the peas for 2-3 minutes, then mix the hot drained peas with the mayo mixture.

3. Add the remaining ingredients then refrigerate before serving.

Nutrition

- Calories: 132

- Total Carbs: 6g

- Net Carbs: 5g

- Protein: 2g

- Potassium: 258mg

- Phosphorous: 64mg

145. Autumn Orzo Salad

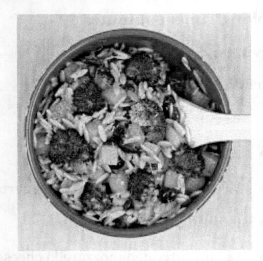

Preparation Time: 1 hour

Cooking Time: 0 minutes

Servings: 4

Ingredients

- 2 cup cooked orzo
- 1 medium apple, cored and diced
- 1 tbsp. fresh basil, chopped
- 2 tbsp. fresh lemon juice
- 2 tbsp. blanched, sliced almonds
- 2 tbsp. extra-virgin olive oil
- ¼ tsp. freshly ground black pepper

Directions

1. Combine all the ingredients except the almonds together in a large bowl.

2. Refrigerate for 3 minutes.

3. Sprinkle with the almonds when you are ready to serve.

Nutrition

- Calories: 227
- Total Carbs: 29g
- Net Carbs: 26g
- Protein: 5g
- Potassium: 126mg
- Phosphorous: 62mg

146. Pumpkin Bacon Soup

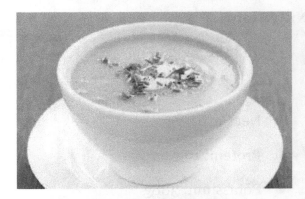

Preparation Time: 10 minutes

Cooking Time: 15 minutes

Servings: 2

Ingredients

- 2 teaspoons ground ginger
- 1 teaspoon cinnamon
- 1 cup applesauce
- 3 ½ cups low sodium chicken broth
- 1 onion, chopped
- 1 slice of bacon

- 1 29-ounce can pumpkin

- Pepper, to taste

- ½ cup light sour cream

Directions

1. Take a medium-large cooking pot; add bacon and cook on both sides over medium heat until crispy for 4-5 minutes.

2. Remove bacon fat.

3. Add ginger, applesauce, chicken broth, pumpkin, and black pepper to taste. Stir mixture.

4. Over low heat, simmer the mixture for about 10 minutes. Season to taste.

5. Take off heat and mix in the cream.

6. Serve warm.

Nutrition

- Calories: 256 Fat: 9g

- Phosphorus: 192mg

- Potassium: 746mg

- Sodium: 148mg Carbohydrates: 33g

- Protein: 8g

147. Chicken Okra Stew

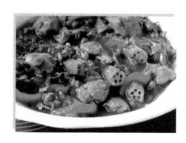

Preparation Time: 10 minutes

Cooking Time: 25 minutes

Servings: 6

Ingredients

- 1 cup sliced onions

- ¾ cup green peppers

- 2 cloves garlic, minced

- 3 tablespoons vegetable oil

- 2 pounds chicken breasts, cut in bite-size pieces

- 1 10-ounce bag frozen carrots

- ¼ teaspoon dried basil

- ¼ teaspoon black pepper

- 2 tablespoons all-purpose flour

- 2 10 ½-ounce cans low-sodium chicken broth

- 6 pounds sliced okra

Directions

1. Take a medium-large cooking pot or Dutch oven, heat 2 tablespoons oil over medium heat.

2. Add chicken and stir-cook until evenly brown. Set aside.

3. Add 1 tablespoon oil. Add onion, garlic, green peppers, and stir-cook until they become softened.

4. Add flour and stir-cook for 2-3 minutes.

5. Add broth, chicken, and boil the mixture.

6. Add carrots, black pepper, and basil.

7. Over low heat, cover, and simmer the mixture for about 10-15 minutes until gravy thickens.

8. Add okra and cook for 5-10 minutes more until tender.

9. Serve with cooked white rice (optional).

Nutrition

- Calories: 153
- Fat: 8g
- Phosphorus: 135mg
- Potassium: 469mg
- Sodium: 110mg
- Carbohydrates: 14g
- Protein: 10g

148. Classic Chicken Soup

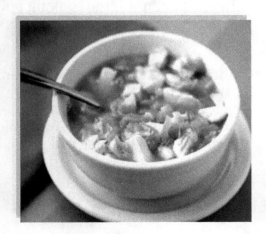

Preparation Time: 10 minutes

Cooking Time: 35 minutes

Servings: 2

Ingredients

- 2 teaspoons minced garlic
- 2 celery stalks, chopped
- 1 tablespoon unsalted butter
- ½ sweet onion, diced
- 1 carrot, diced
- 4 cups of water
- 1 teaspoon chopped fresh thyme
- 2 cups chopped cooked chicken breast
- 1 cup chicken stock
- Black pepper (ground), to taste
- 2 tablespoons chopped fresh parsley

Directions

1. Take a medium-large cooking pot, heat oil over medium heat.

2. Add onion and stir-cook until become translucent and softened.

3. Add garlic and stir-cook until you become fragrant.

4. Add celery, carrot, chicken, chicken stock, and water.

5. Boil the mixture.

6. Over low heat, simmer the mixture for about 25-30 minutes until veggies are tender.

7. Mix in thyme and cook for 2 minutes. Season to taste with black pepper.

8. Serve warm with parsley on top.

Nutrition

- Calories: 135

- Fat: 6g

- Phosphorus: 122mg

- Potassium: 208mg

- Sodium: 74mg

- Carbohydrates: 3g

- Protein: 15g

149. Beef Okra Soup

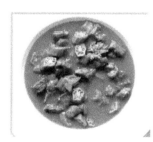

Preparation Time: 10 minutes

Cooking Time: 45 minutes

Servings: 5

Ingredients

- ½ cup okra

- ½ teaspoon basil

- ½ cup carrots, diced

- 3 ½ cups water

- 1 pound beef stew meat

- 1 cup raw sliced onions

- ½ cup green peas

- 1 teaspoon black pepper

- ½ teaspoon thyme

- ½ cup corn kernels

Directions

1. Take a medium-large cooking pot, heat oil over medium heat.

2. Add water, beef stew meat, black pepper, onions, basil, thyme, and stir-cook for 40-45 minutes until meat is tender.

3. Add all veggies. Over low heat, simmer the mixture for about 20-25 minutes. Add more water if needed.

4. Serve soup warm.

Nutrition

- Calories: 187

- Fat: 12g

- Phosphorus: 119mg

- Potassium: 288mg

- Sodium: 59mg

- Carbohydrates: 7g

- Protein: 11g

150. Green Bean Veggie Stew

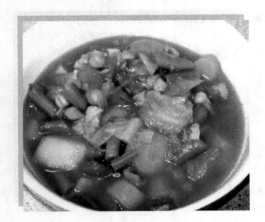

Preparation Time: 10 minutes

Cooking Time: 35 minutes

Servings: 2

Ingredients

- 6 cups shredded green cabbage
- 3 celery stalks, chopped
- 1 teaspoon unsalted butter
- ½ large sweet onion, chopped
- 1 teaspoon minced garlic
- 1 scallion, chopped
- 2 tablespoons chopped fresh parsley
- 2 tablespoons lemon juice
- 1 teaspoon chopped fresh oregano
- 1 tablespoon chopped fresh thyme
- 1 teaspoon chopped savory
- Water
- 1 cup fresh green beans, cut into 1-inch pieces

- Black pepper (ground), to taste

Directions

1. Take a medium-large cooking pot, heat butter over medium heat.

2. Add onion and stir-cook until become translucent and softened.

3. Add garlic and stir-cook until you become fragrant.

4. Add cabbage, celery, scallion, parsley, lemon juice, thyme, savory, and oregano; add water to cover veggies by 3-4 inches.

5. Stir the mixture and boil it.

6. Over low heat, cover, and simmer the mixture for about 25 minutes until veggies are tender.

7. Add green beans and cook for 2-3 more minutes. Season with black pepper to taste.

8. Serve warm.

Nutrition

- Calories: 56
- Fat: 1g
- Phosphorus: 36mg
- Potassium: 194mg
- Sodium: 31mg
- Carbohydrates: 7g
- Protein: 1g

151. Chicken Pasta Soup

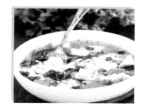

Preparation Time: 10 minutes

Cooking Time: 20 minutes

Servings: 6

Ingredients

- 1 ½ cups baby spinach

- 2 tablespoons orzo (tiny pasta)

- 1 tablespoon dry white wine

- 1 14-ounce low sodium chicken broth

- 2 plum tomatoes, chopped

- ½ teaspoon Italian seasoning

- 1 large shallot, chopped

- 1 small zucchini, diced

- 8ounces chicken tenders

- 1 tablespoon extra-virgin olive oil

Directions

1. Take a medium saucepan or skillet, add oil. Heat over medium heat.

2. Add chicken and stir-cook for 3 minutes until evenly brown. Set aside.

3. In the pan, add zucchini, Italian seasoning, shallot; stir-cook until veggies are softened.

4. Add tomatoes, wine, broth, and orzo.

5. Boil the mixture.

6. Over low heat, cover, and simmer the mixture for about 3 minutes.

7. Mix in spinach and cooked chicken; stir and serve warm.

Nutrition

- Calories: 103 Fat: 3g

- Phosphorus: 125mg

- Potassium: 264mg

- Sodium: 84mg Carbohydrates: 6g

- Protein: 12g

152. Herbed Cabbage Stew

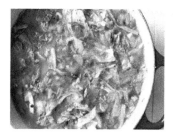

Preparation Time: 20 minutes

Cooking Time: 35 minutes

Servings: 2

Ingredients

- 1 teaspoon unsalted butter

- ½ large sweet onion, chopped

- 1 teaspoon minced garlic

- 6 cups shredded green cabbage

- 3 celery stalks, chopped with the leafy tops

- 1 scallion, both green and white parts, chopped

- 2 tablespoons chopped fresh parsley

- 2 tablespoons freshly squeezed lemon juice

- 1 tablespoon chopped fresh thyme

- 1 teaspoon chopped savory

- 1 teaspoon chopped fresh oregano

- Water

- Green beans, 1 cup, chopped

- Freshly ground black pepper

Directions

1. In a medium stockpot over medium-high heat, melt the butter. Sauté the onion and garlic in the melted butter for about 3 minutes or until the vegetables are softened. Add the cabbage, celery, scallion, parsley, lemon juice, thyme, savory, and oregano to the pot, and add enough water to cover the vegetables by about 4 inches.

2. Bring the soup to a boil, reduce the heat to low, and simmer the soup for about 25 minutes or until the vegetables are tender. Add the green beans and simmer 3 minutes. Season with pepper.

Nutrition

- Calories: 33

- Fat: 1g

- Carbs: 6g

- Phosphorus: 29mg

- Potassium: 187mg

- Sodium: 20mg

- Protein: 1g

153. French Onion Soup

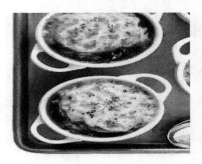

Preparation Time: 20 minutes

Cooking Time: 50 minutes

Servings: 3

Ingredients

- 2 tablespoons unsalted butter

- 4 Vidalia onions, sliced thin

- 2 cups Easy Chicken Stock (here)

- 2 cups water

- 1 tablespoon chopped fresh thyme

- Freshly ground black pepper

Directions

1. Set your butter on to melt in a saucepan on medium heat. Add the onions to the saucepan and cook

them slowly, stirring frequently, for about 30 minutes or until the onions are caramelized and tender.

2. Add the chicken stock and water and bring the soup to a boil. Switch to low heat to simmer for 15 minutes. Stir in the thyme and season the soup with pepper. Serve piping hot.

Nutrition

- Calories: 90

- Fat: 6g

- Carbs: 7g

- Phosphorus: 22mg

- Potassium: 192mg

- Sodium: 57mg

- Protein: 2g

154. Creamy Broccoli Soup

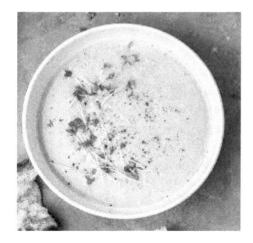

Preparation Time: 10 minutes

Cooking Time: 15 minutes

Servings: 4

Ingredients

- 1 teaspoon extra-virgin olive oil

- ½ sweet onion, roughly chopped

- 2 cups chopped broccoli

- 4 cups low-sodium vegetable broth

- Freshly ground black pepper

- 1 cup Homemade Rice Milk or unsweetened store-bought rice milk

- ¼ cup grated Parmesan cheese

Directions

1. In a medium saucepan over medium-high heat, heat the olive oil. Add the onion and cook for 3 to 5 minutes, until it begins to soften. Add the broccoli and broth, and season with pepper.

2. Bring to a boil, reduce the heat, and simmer uncovered for 10 minutes, until the broccoli is just tender but still bright green. Transfer the soup mixture to a blender. Add the rice milk, and process until smooth. Return to the saucepan, stir in the Parmesan cheese, and serve.

Nutrition

- Calories: 88

- Fat: 3g Carbs: 12g

- Protein: 4g Phosphorus: 87mg

- Potassium: 201mg

- Sodium: 281mg

155. Cream of Watercress Soup

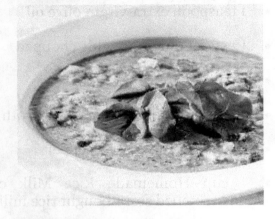

Preparation Time: 15 minutes

Cooking Time: 1 hour 15 minutes

Servings: 4

Ingredients

- 6 garlic cloves

- ½ teaspoon olive oil

- 1 teaspoon unsalted butter

- ½ sweet onion, chopped

- 4 cups chopped watercress

- ¼ cup chopped fresh parsley

- 3 cups water

- ¼ cup heavy cream

- 1 tablespoon freshly squeezed lemon juice

- Freshly ground black pepper

Directions

1. Preheat the oven to 400°F. Set your garlic on a sheet of foil. Drizzle with olive oil and fold the foil into a little packet. Place the packet in a pie plate and roast the garlic for about 20 minutes or until very soft.

2. Switch off the oven and set your garlic to cool. Add your butter to melt in a saucepan on medium heat. Sauté the onion for about 4 minutes or until soft. Add the watercress and parsley; sauté 5 minutes. Stir in the water and roasted garlic pulp. Allow to boil then switch the heat to low.

3. Simmer the soup for about 20 minutes or until the vegetables are soft. Cool the soup for about 5 minutes, then purée in batches in a food processor (or use a large bowl and a handheld immersion blender), along with the heavy cream.

4. Transfer the soup to the pot, and set over low heat until warmed through. Add the lemon juice and season with pepper.

Nutrition

- Calories: 97

- Fat: 8g

- Carbs: 5g

- Phosphorus: 46mg

- Potassium: 198mg

- Sodium: 23mg

- Protein: 2g

156. Curried Cauliflower Soup

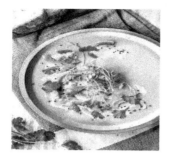

Preparation Time: 20 minutes

Cooking Time: 30 minutes

Servings: 6

Ingredients

- 1 teaspoon unsalted butter

- 1 small sweet onion, chopped

- 2 teaspoons minced garlic

- 1 small head cauliflower, cut into small florets

- 3 cups water, or more to cover the cauliflower

- 2 teaspoons curry powder

- ½ cup light sour cream

- 3 tablespoons chopped fresh cilantro

Directions

1. In a large saucepan, heat the butter over medium-high heat and sauté the onion and garlic for about 3 minutes or until softened. Add the cauliflower, water, and curry powder.

2. Bring the soup to a boil, then reduce the heat to low and simmer for about 20 minutes or until the cauliflower is tender. Pour the soup into a food processor and purée until the soup is smooth and creamy (or use a large bowl and a handheld immersion blender).

3. Transfer the soup back into a saucepan and stir in the sour cream and cilantro. Heat the soup on medium-low for about 5 minutes or until warmed through.

Nutrition

- Calories: 33 Fat: 2g

- Carbs: 4g Phosphorus: 30mg

- Potassium: 167mg

- Sodium: 22mg Protein: 1g

157. Asparagus Lemon Soup

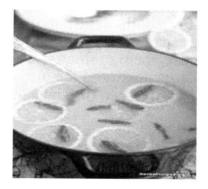

Preparation Time: 10 minutes

Cooking Time: 25 minutes

Servings: 4

Ingredients

- 1 pound asparagus

- 2 tablespoons extra-virgin olive oil

- ½ sweet onion, chopped

- 4 cups low-sodium chicken stock

- ½ cup Homemade Rice Milk or unsweetened store-bought rice milk

- Freshly ground black pepper

- Juice of 1 lemon

Directions

1. Cut the asparagus tips from the spears and set aside. In a small stockpot over medium heat, heat the olive oil. Add the onion and cook, stirring frequently for 3 to 5 minutes, until it begins to soften. Add the stock and asparagus stalks, and bring to a boil.

2. Reduce the heat and simmer until the asparagus is tender, about 15 minutes. Transfer to a blender or food processor, and carefully purée until smooth. Return to the pot, add the asparagus tips, and simmer until tender, about 5 minutes. Add the rice milk, pepper, and lemon juice, and stir until heated through. Serve.

Nutrition

- Calories: 145

- Fat: 9g

- Carbs: 13g

- Protein: 8g

- Phosphorus: 143mg

- Potassium: 497mg

- Sodium: 92mg

158. Roasted Red Pepper and Eggplant Soup

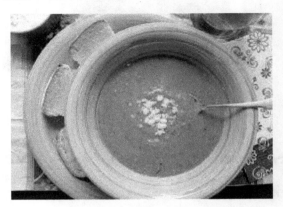

Preparation Time: 20 minutes

Cooking Time: 40 minutes

Servings: 2

Ingredients

- 1 small sweet onion, cut into quarters

- 2 small red bell peppers, halved

- 2 cups cubed eggplant

- 2 garlic cloves, crushed

- 1 tablespoon olive oil

- 1 cup Easy Chicken Stock

- Water

- ¼ cup chopped fresh basil

- Freshly ground black pepper

Directions

1. Preheat the oven to 350°F. Put the onions, red peppers, eggplant, and garlic in a large ovenproof baking dish. Drizzle the vegetables with the olive oil. Roast the vegetables for

about 30 minutes or until they are slightly charred and soft.

2. Cool the vegetables slightly and remove the skin from the peppers. Purée the vegetables in batches in a food processor (or in a large bowl, using a handheld immersion blender) with the chicken stock.

3. Transfer the soup to a medium pot and add enough water to reach the desired thickness. Heat the soup to a simmer and add the basil. Season with pepper and serve.

Nutrition

- Calories: 61 Fat: 2g Carbs: 9g

- Phosphorus: 33mg

- Potassium: 198mg

- Sodium: 95mg Protein: 2g

159. Curried Carrot and Beet Soup

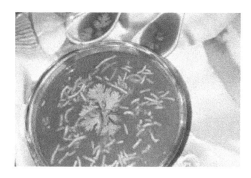

Preparation Time: 10 minutes

Cooking Time: 50 minutes

Servings: 4

Ingredients

- 1 large red beet

- 5 carrots, chopped

- 1 tablespoon curry powder

- 3 cups Homemade Rice Milk or unsweetened store-bought rice milk

- Freshly ground black pepper

- Yogurt, for serving

Directions

1. Preheat the oven to 400°F.Wrap the beet in aluminum foil and roast for 45 minutes, until the vegetable is tender when pierced with a fork. Remove from the oven and let cool. In a saucepan, add the carrots and cover with water. Bring to a boil, reduce the heat, cover, and simmer for 10 minutes, until tender.

2. Transfer the carrots and beet to a food processor, and process until smooth. Add the curry powder and rice milk. Season with pepper. Serve topped with a dollop of yogurt.

Nutrition

- Calories: 112

- Fat: 1g

- Carbs: 24g

- Fiber: 7g

- Protein: 3g

- Phosphorus: 57mg

- Potassium: 468mg

- Sodium: 129mg

160. Winter Chicken Stew

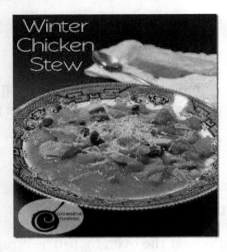

Preparation Time: 10 minutes

Cooking Time: 50 minutes

Servings: 4

Ingredients

- 1 tablespoon olive oil

- Chicken thighs, skinless, boneless, cubed

- ½ sweet onion, chopped

- 1 tablespoon minced garlic

- 2 cups Easy Chicken Stock

- 1 cup plus 2 tablespoons water

- 1 carrot, sliced

- 2 celery stalks, sliced

- 1 turnip, sliced thin

- 1 tablespoon chopped fresh thyme

- 1 teaspoon finely chopped fresh rosemary

- 2 teaspoons cornstarch

- Freshly ground black pepper

Directions

1. Place a large saucepan on medium-high heat and add the olive oil. Sauté the chicken for about 6 minutes or until it is lightly browned, stirring often. Add the onion and garlic and sauté for 3 minutes. Add the chicken stock, 1 cup water, carrot, celery, and turnip and bring the stew to a boil.

2. Reduce the heat to low and simmer for about 30 minutes or until the chicken is cooked through and tender. Add the thyme and rosemary and simmer for 3 more minutes. In a small bowl, stir together the 2 tablespoons water and the cornstarch, and add the mixture to the stew. Stir to incorporate the cornstarch mixture and cook for 3 to 4 minutes or until the stew thickens. Remove from the heat and season with pepper.

Nutrition

- Calories: 141

- Fat: 8g

- Carbs: 5g

- Phosphorus: 53mg

- Potassium: 192mg

- Sodium: 214mg

- Protein: 9g

161. Turkey Burger Soup

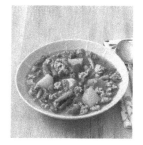

Preparation Time: 10 minutes

Cooking Time: 25 minutes

Servings: 6

Ingredients

- 2 tablespoons extra-virgin olive oil

- 1 pound ground turkey breast

- ½ sweet onion, chopped

- 3 garlic cloves, minced

- Freshly ground black pepper

- 1 (16-ounce) can low-sodium diced tomatoes, drained

- 4 cups Simple Chicken Broth or low-sodium store-bought chicken stock

- 1 cup sliced carrots

- 1 cup sliced celery

- 1 tablespoon chopped fresh basil

- 1 tablespoon chopped fresh oregano

- 1 tablespoon chopped fresh thyme

Directions

1. In a medium stockpot over medium-high heat, heat the olive oil. Add the turkey, onion, and garlic, and cook, stirring frequently, until the turkey is browned. Season with pepper. Reduce the heat to low, and simmer for 20 minutes. Serve.

Nutrition

- Calories: 260

- Fat: 9g

- Carbs: 19g

- Protein: 29g

- Phosphorus: 106mg

- Potassium: 449mg

- Sodium: 296mg

161. Salmon Cucumber Salad

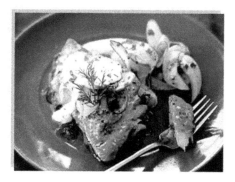

Preparation Time: 10 minutes

Cooking Time: 10 minutes

Servings: 2

Ingredients

- 1 cup diced fennel bulb

- 1 cup diced red onions

- ½ pound salmon fillets

- 1 cup cucumber, peeled and diced

- 2 tablespoons + 1 teaspoon olive oil

- 3 tablespoons apple cider vinegar

- Black pepper, to taste

Directions

1. Preheat an oven to 400⁰F. Grease a baking dish with 1 teaspoon olive oil.

2. Season salmon with black pepper with skin side down.

3. Placed over the baking dish, bake for 8-10 minutes until easy to flake.

4. Flake salmon and add it in a bowl.

5. In another bowl, whisk vinegar and remaining oil.

6. Add the salmon and combine it. Add remaining ingredients and combine well.

7. Serve fresh.

Nutrition

- Calories: 288

- Fat: 14g

- Phosphorus: 217mg

- Potassium: 548mg

- Sodium: 178mg

- Carbohydrates: 17g

- Protein: 26g

162. Shrimp Mayo Salad

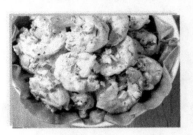

Preparation Time: 40 minutes

Cooking Time: 0 minutes

Servings: 2

Ingredients

- 1 tablespoon celery, chopped

- 1 tablespoon green pepper, chopped

- 1 tablespoon onion, chopped

- 1 pound shrimp, boiled, chopped and deveined

- 1 hard-boiled egg, chopped

- 1 teaspoon lemon juice

- ½ teaspoon chili powder

- ⅛ Teaspoon Tabasco or hot sauce

- 2 tablespoons mayonnaise

- ½ teaspoon dry mustard lettuce, chopped or shredded (optional)

- Lettuce leaves

Directions

1. In a mixing bowl, add all ingredients except lettuce. Combine to mix well with each other.

2. Refrigerate for 30 minutes.

3. Arrange lettuce leaves on a plate; add salad mixture on top.

4. Serve fresh.

Nutrition

- Calories: 161 Fat: 5g

- Phosphorus: 271mg

- Potassium: 224mg

- Sodium: 255mg Carbohydrates: 2g

- Protein: 26g

163. Beet Feta Salad

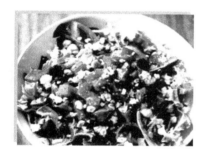

Preparation Time: 10 minutes

Cooking Time: 30 minutes

Servings: 5

Ingredients

- 4 cups baby salad greens

- ½ sweet onion, sliced

- 8 small beets, trimmed

- 2 tablespoons + 1 teaspoon extra-virgin olive oil

- 1 tablespoon white wine vinegar

- 1 teaspoon Dijon mustard

- Black pepper (ground), to taste

- 2 tablespoons crumbled feta cheese

- 2 tablespoons walnut pieces

Directions

1. Preheat an oven to 400°F. Grease an aluminum foil with some cooking spray.

2. Add beets with 1 teaspoon of olive oil; combine and wrap foil.

3. Bake for 30 minutes until it becomes tender. Cut beets into wedges.

4. In a mixing bowl, add remaining olive oil, vinegar, black pepper, and mustard. Combine to mix well with each other.

5. In a mixing bowl, add salad greens, onion, feta cheese, and walnuts. Combine to mix well with each other.

6. Add half of the prepared vinaigrette and toss well.

7. Add beet and combine well.

8. Drizzle remaining vinaigrette and serve fresh.

Nutrition

- Calories: 184 Fat: 9g

- Phosphorus: 98mg

- Potassium: 601mg

- Sodium: 235mg Carbohydrates: 19g

- Protein: 4g

164. Cabbage Pear Salad

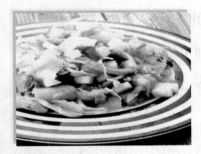

Preparation Time: 10 minutes + 1 hour

Cooking Time: 0 minutes

Servings: 6

Ingredients

- 2 scallions, chopped
- 2 cups finely shredded green cabbage
- 1 cup finely shredded red cabbage
- ½ red bell pepper, boiled and chopped
- ½ cup chopped cilantro
- 2 celery stalks, chopped
- 1 Asian pear, cored and grated
- ¼ cup olive oil
- Juice of 1 lime
- Zest of 1 lime
- 1 teaspoon granulated sugar

Directions

1. In a mixing bowl, add cabbages, scallions, celery, pear, red pepper, and cilantro. Combine to mix well with each other.
2. Take another mixing bowl; add olive oil, lime juice, lime zest, and sugar. Combine to mix well with each other.
3. Add dressing over and toss well.
4. Refrigerate for 1 hour; serve chilled.

Nutrition

- Calories: 128 Fat: 8g
- Phosphorus: 25mg
- Potassium: 149mg
- Sodium: 57mg Carbohydrates: 2g
- Protein: 6g

165. Arugula Parmesan Salad

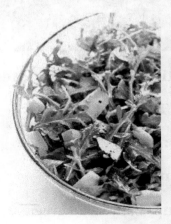

Preparation Time: 10 minutes

Cooking Time: 0 minutes

Servings: 4

Ingredients

- 2 cups loosely packed arugula

- 1 tablespoon extra-virgin olive oil

- 1 shallot, thinly sliced

- 3 celery stalks, cut into 1-inch pieces about ¼ inch thick

- 2 tablespoons white wine vinegar

- Black pepper (ground), to taste

- 2 tablespoons Parmesan cheese, grated

Directions

1. In a mixing bowl, add shallot, celery stalks, and arugula. Combine to mix well with each other.

2. Take another mixing bowl; add olive oil, vinegar, and black pepper. Combine to mix well with each other.

3. Add dressing over and toss well.

4. Add cheese on top, and serve fresh.

Nutrition

- Calories: 61

- Fat: 4g

- Phosphorus: 34mg

- Potassium: 53mg

- Sodium: 55mg

- Carbohydrates: 1g

- Protein: 2g

166. Cabbage Turkey Soup

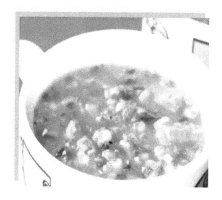

Preparation Time: 10 minutes

Cooking Time: 45 minutes

Servings: 6

Ingredients

- ½ cup shredded green cabbage

- ½ cup bulgur

- 2 dried bay leaves

- 2 tablespoons chopped fresh parsley

- 1 teaspoon chopped fresh sage

- 1 teaspoon chopped fresh thyme

- 1 celery stalk, chopped

- 1 carrot, sliced thin

- ½ sweet onion, chopped

- 1 teaspoon minced garlic

- 1 teaspoon olive oil

- ½ pound cooked ground turkey, 93% lean

- 4 cups of water

- 1 cup chicken stock

- Pinch red pepper flakes

- Black pepper (ground), to taste

Directions

1. Take a large saucepan or cooking pot, add oil. Heat over medium heat.

2. Add turkey and stir-cook for 4-5 minutes until evenly brown.

3. Add onion and garlic and sauté for about 3 minutes to soften veggies.

4. Add water, chicken stock, cabbage, bulgur, celery, carrot, and bay leaves.

5. Boil the mixture.

6. Over low heat, cover, and simmer the mixture for about 30-35 minutes until bulgur is cooked well and tender.

7. Remove bay leaves. Add parsley, sage, thyme, and red pepper flakes; stir mixture and season with black pepper.

8. Serve warm.

Nutrition

- Calories: 83

- Fat: 4g

- Phosphorus: 91mg

- Potassium: 185mg

- Sodium: 63mg

- Carbohydrates: 2g

- Protein: 8g

167. Classic Onion Soup

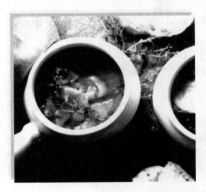

Preparation Time: 10 minutes

Cooking Time: 45 minutes

Servings: 4

Ingredients

- 2cups chicken stock

- 2 cups of water

- 2 tablespoons unsalted butter

- 4 Vidalia onions, sliced thin

- 1 tablespoon chopped fresh thyme

- Black pepper (ground), to taste

Directions

1. Take a medium-large cooking pot or saucepan, heat butter over medium heat.

2. Add onion and stir-cook until become caramelized and softened, about 30 seconds.

3. Add chicken stock and water.

4. Boil the mixture.

5. Over low heat, simmer the mixture for about 15 minutes.

6. Add thyme and season with pepper.

7. Stir and serve warm.

Nutrition

- Calories: 104 Fat: 6g

- Phosphorus: 28mg

- Potassium: 188mg

- Sodium: 61mg Carbohydrates: 6g

- Protein: 2g

168. Chicken Noodle Soup

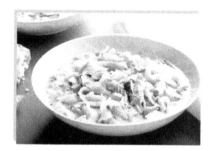

Preparation Time: 10 minutes

Cooking Time: 45 minutes

Servings: 6

Ingredients

- 2 tablespoons vegetable oil

- 1 cup egg noodles

- 1 teaspoon black pepper

- 1 teaspoon caraway seed

- 3 ½ cups water

- 1 pound chicken parts

- 1 teaspoon red pepper

- ¼ cup lemon juice

- 1 tablespoon poultry seasoning

- 1 teaspoon sugar

- 1 teaspoon garlic powder

- 1 teaspoon oregano

- ½ cup celery

- 1 teaspoon onion powder

- ½ cup green pepper

Directions

1. Coat chicken pieces with lemon juice.

2. Take a medium-large cooking pot, add chicken, water, garlic powder, poultry seasoning, black pepper, onion powder, vegetable oil, caraway seed, oregano, red pepper, and sugar.

3. Stir mixture and heat over medium heat for 25-30 minutes until chicken is tender. Add other ingredients; stir and continue to cook for 15 minutes more. Add more water if needed.

4. Serve warm.

Nutrition

- Calories: 118 Fat: 8g

- Phosphorus: 41mg

- Potassium: 104mg

- Sodium: 21mg Carbohydrates: 6g

- Protein: 3g

169. Asian Cabbage Slaw

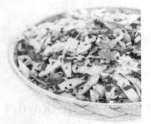

Preparation Time: 10 minutes

Cooking Time: 0 minutes

Servings: 4

Ingredients

- 4 cup shredded cabbage
- ¼ cup canned, sliced water chestnuts
- 3 green onions, finely diced
- 1 tbsp. sesame seeds
- ½ cup chow Mein noodles
- 2 tbsp. canola oil
- 2 tbsp. apple cider vinegar
- 2 tsp. sugar
- ¼ tsp. black pepper

Directions

1. Place vegetables and sesame seeds in a large bowl.
2. Dissolve sugar in vinegar in a small bowl.
3. Whisk in the oil.
4. Pour the dressing over the cabbage and mix until thoroughly combined.
5. Chill for several hours or overnight.
6. Add chow Mein noodles and toss before serving.

Nutrition

- Calories: 130
- Total Carbs: 8g
- Net Carbs: 5g
- Protein: 2g
- Potassium: 183mg
- Phosphorous: 50mg

170. Carrot and Lemon Salad

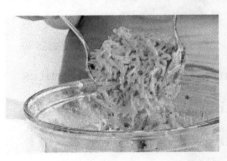

Preparation Time: 1 hour 10 minutes

Cooking Time: 0 minutes

Servings: 4

Ingredients

- 4 cup fresh carrots
- 5 lemons
- ½ cup granulated sugar

Directions

1. Shred carrots in a food processor.

2. Wash the lemons and remove the tips. Roughly chop the lemon and add to the food processor with carrots.

3. Stir in the sugar and chill in the refrigerator for one hour before serving.

Nutrition

- Calories: 68

- Total Carbs: 16g

- Net Carbs: 12g

- Protein: 1g

- Potassium: 220mg

- Phosphorous: 17mg

CHAPTER 9:

Dessert Recipes

171. Cheesecake Bites

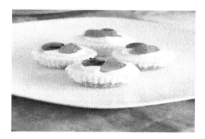

Preparation Time: 10 minutes

Cooking Time: 5 minutes

Servings: 16

Ingredients

- 8 oz. cream cheese

- 1/2 tsp. vanilla

- 1/4 cup swerve

Directions

1. Add all ingredients into the mixing bowl and blend until well combined.

2. Place bowl into the fridge for 1 hour.

3. Remove bowl from the fridge. Make small balls from cheese mixture and place them on a baking dish.

4. Serve and enjoy.

Nutrition

- Calories 50 Fat 4.9 g

- Carbohydrates 0.4 g

- Sugar 0.1 g Protein 1.1 g

- Cholesterol 16 mg

172. Pumpkin Bites

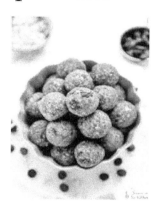

Preparation Time: 10 minutes

Cooking Time: 5 minutes

Servings: 12

Ingredients

- 8 oz. cream cheese

- 1 tsp. vanilla

- 1 tsp. pumpkin pie spice
- 1/4 cup coconut flour
- 1/4 cup erythritol
- 1/2 cup pumpkin puree
- 4 oz. butter

Directions

1. Add all ingredients into the mixing bowl and beat using a hand mixer until well combined.
2. Scoop mixture into the silicone ice cube tray and place it in the refrigerator until set.
3. Serve and enjoy.

Nutrition

- Calories: 149 Fat: 14.6 g
- Carbohydrates: 8.1 g
- Sugar: 5.4 g Protein: 2 g
- Cholesterol: 41 mg
-

173. Protein Balls

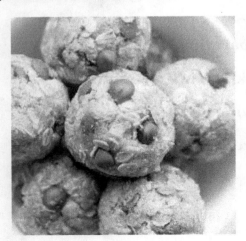

Preparation Time: 5 minutes

Cooking Time: 5 minutes

Servings: 12

Ingredients

- 3/4 cup peanut butter
- 1 tsp. cinnamon
- 3 tbsp. erythritol
- 1 1/2 cup almond flour

Directions

1. Add all ingredients into the mixing bowl and blend until well combined.
2. Place bowl into the fridge for 30 minutes.
3. Remove bowl from the fridge. Make small balls from mixture and place on a baking dish.
4. Serve and enjoy.

Nutrition

- Calories: 179
- Fat: 14.8g
- Carbohydrates: 10.1g
- Sugar: 5.3g
- Protein: 7g
- Cholesterol: 0mg

174. Cashew Cheese Bites

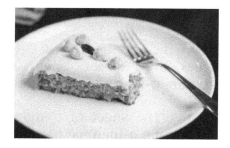

Preparation Time: 5 minutes

Cooking Time: 5 minutes

Servings: 12

Ingredients

- 8 oz. cream cheese
- 1 tsp. cinnamon
- 1 cup cashew butter

Directions

1. Add all ingredients into the blender and blend until smooth.
2. Pour blended mixture into the mini muffin liners and place them in the refrigerator until set.
3. Serve and enjoy.

Nutrition

- Calories: 192
- Fat: 17.1g
- Carbohydrates: 6.5g
- Sugar: 0g
- Protein: 5.2g
- Cholesterol: 21mg

175. Healthy Cinnamon Lemon Tea

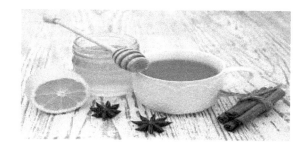

Preparation Time: 5 minutes

Cooking Time: 5 minutes

Servings: 1

Ingredients

- 1/2 tbsp. fresh lemon juice
- 1 cup of water
- 1 tsp. ground cinnamon

Directions

1. Add water in a saucepan and bring to boil over medium heat.
2. Add cinnamon and stir to cinnamon dissolve.
3. Add lemon juice and stir well.
4. Serve hot.

Nutrition

- Calories: 9 Fat: 0.2g
- Carbohydrates: 2g
- Sugar: 0.3g Protein: 0.2g
- Cholesterol: 0mg

176. Apple Pie

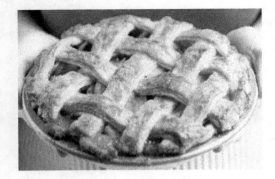

Preparation time: 10 minutes

Cooking time: 50 minutes

Servings: 6

Ingredients

- 6 medium apples, peeled, cored & sliced

- 1/2 cup granulated sugar

- 1 tsp. ground cinnamon

- 6 tbsp. butter

- 2-2/3 cups all-purpose flour

- 1 cup shortening

- 6 tbsp. water

Directions

1. Preheat your oven to 425 degrees F.

2. Toss the apple slices with cinnamon and sugar in a bowl and set it aside covered.

3. Blend the flour with the shortening in a pastry blender then add chilled water by the tablespoon.

4. Continue mixing and adding the water until it forms a smooth dough ball.

5. Divide the dough into two equal-size pieces and spread them into 2 separate 9-inch sheets.

6. Arrange the sheet of dough at the bottom of a 9-inch pie pan.

7. Spread the apples in the pie shell and spread a tablespoon of butter over it.

8. Cover the filling with the remaining sheet of the dough and pinch down the edges.

9. Carve 1-inch cuts on top of the pie and bake for 50 minutes or more until golden.

10. Slice and serve.

Nutrition

- Calories: 517

- Protein: 4g

- Carbohydrates: 51g

- Fat: 33g

- Cholesterol: 24mg

- Sodium: 65mg

- Potassium: 145mg

- Phosphorus: 43mg

- Calcium: 24mg

- Fiber: 2.7g

177. Banana Pudding Dessert

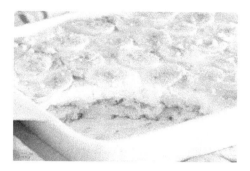

Preparation time: 10 minutes

Cooking time: 5 minutes

Servings: 4

Ingredients

- 12 oz. vanilla wafers

- 2 boxes banana cream pudding mix

- 2-1/2 cups unenriched rice milk

- 8 oz. dairy whipped topping

Directions

1. Line the bottom of a 9x13 inch pan with a layer of wafers.

2. Mix the banana pudding mix with 2.5 cups of milk in a saucepan.

3. Bring it to a boil while constantly stirring.

4. Pour this banana pudding over the wafers.

5. Add another layer of wafers over the pudding layer and press them down gently.

6. Place the layered pudding in the refrigerator for 1 hour.

7. Garnish with whipped cream and serve.

Nutrition

- Calories: 259 Protein: 3g

- Carbohydrates: 46g

- Fat: 7g Cholesterol: 3mg

- Sodium: 276mg

- Potassium: 52mg

- Phosphorus: 40mg

- Calcium: 9mg Fiber: 0.3g

178. Blueberry Cream Cones

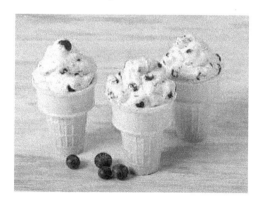

Preparation time: 10 minutes

Cooking time: 0 minutes

Servings: 6

Ingredients

- 4 oz. cream cheese

- 1-1/2 cup whipped topping

- 1-1/4 cup fresh or frozen blueberries

- 1/4 cup blueberry jam or preserves

- 6 small ice cream cones

Directions

1. Start by softening the cream cheese then beat it in a mixer until fluffy.

2. Fold in jam and fruits.

3. Divide the mixture into the ice cream cones.

4. Serve fresh.

Nutrition

- Calories: 177 Protein: 3g

- Carbohydrates: 21g

- Cholesterol: 21mg

- Sodium: 95mg

- Potassium: 81mg

- Phosphorus: 40mg

- Calcium: 24mg Fiber: 1.0g

179. Spiced Peaches

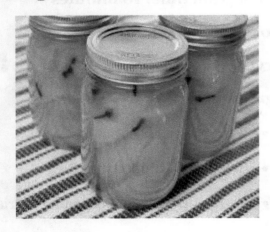

Preparation Time: 5 minutes

Cooking Time: 10 minutes

Servings: 2

Ingredients

- Canned peaches with juices – 1 cup

- Cornstarch – ½ teaspoon

- Ground cloves – 1 teaspoon

- Ground cinnamon – 1 teaspoon

- Ground nutmeg – 1 teaspoon

- Zest of ½ lemon

- Water – ½ cup

Directions

1. Drain peaches.

2. Combine cinnamon, cornstarch, nutmeg, ground cloves, and lemon zest in a pan on the stove.

3. Heat on a medium heat and add peaches.

4. Bring to a boil, reduce the heat and simmer for 10 minutes.

5. Serve.

Nutrition

- Calories: 70 Fat: 0g

- Carb: 14g Phosphorus: 23mg

- Potassium: 176mg

- Sodium: 3mg

- Protein: 1g

180. Cherry Dessert

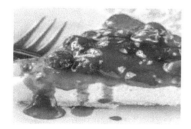

Preparation time: 10 minutes

Cooking time: 20 minutes

Servings: 6

Ingredients

- 1 small package sugar-free cherry gelatin
- 1 pie crust, 9-inch size
- 8 oz. light cream cheese
- 12 oz. whipped topping
- 20 oz. cherry pie filling

Directions

1. Prepare the cherry gelatin as per the given instructions on the packet.
2. Pour the mixture in an 8x8 inch pan and refrigerate until set.
3. Soften the cream cheese at room temperature.
4. Place the 9-inch pie crust in a pie pan and bake it until golden brown.
5. Vigorously, beat the cream cheese in a mixer until fluffy and fold in whipped topping.
6. Dice the gelatin into cubes and add them to the cream cheese mixture.
7. Mix gently then add this mixture to the baking pie shell.
8. Top the cream cheese filling with cherry pie filling.
9. Refrigerate for 3 hours then slice to serve.

Nutrition

- Calories: 258 Protein: 5g
- Carbohydrates: 28g
- Fat: 13g Cholesterol: 11mg
- Sodium: 214mg
- Potassium: 150mg
- Phosphorus: 50mg
- Calcium: 30mg Fiber: 1.0

181. Crunchy Peppermint Cookies

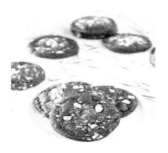

Preparation time: 10 minutes

Cooking time: 12 minutes

Servings: 6

Ingredients

- 1/2 cup unsalted butter

- 18 peppermint candies
- 3/4 cup sugar
- 1 large egg
- 1/4 tsp. peppermint extract
- 1-1/2 cups all-purpose flour
- 1 tsp. baking powder

Directions

1. Soften the butter at room temperature.

2. Add 12 peppermint candies to a zip lock bag and crush them using a mallet.

3. Beat butter with egg, sugar and peppermint extract in a mixer until fluffy.

4. Stir in baking powder and flour and mix well until smooth.

5. Stir in crushed peppermint candies and refrigerate the dough for 1 hour.

6. Meanwhile, layer a baking sheet with parchment paper.

7. Preheat the oven to 350 degrees F.

8. Crush the remaining candies and keep them aside.

9. Make ¾-inch balls out of the dough and place them on the baking sheet.

10. Sprinkle the crushed candies over the balls.

11. Bake them for 12 minutes until slightly browned.

12. Serve fresh and enjoy.

Nutrition

- Calories:150
- Protein: 2g
- Carbohydrates: 22g
- Fat: 6g
- Cholesterol: 24mg
- Sodium: 67mg
- Potassium: 17mg
- Phosphorus: 24mg
- Calcium: 20mg

182. Cranberries Snow

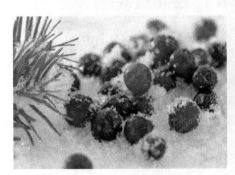

Preparation time: 10 minutes

Cooking time: 12 minutes

Servings: 4

Ingredients

- 1 cup cram-cherry juice
- 12 oz. fresh cranberries
- 2 packets gelatin
- 2 cups granulated sugar

- 1 cup crushed pineapple, canned in juice

- 8 oz. cream cheese

- 3 cups whipped topping

Directions

1. Boil the cram-cherry juice in a saucepan.

2. Stir in cranberries and cook for 12 minutes.

3. Remove the pan from the stove heat and add 1 ¼ cup sugar and gelatin.

4. Mix well until dissolved then allow it to cool for 30 minutes.

5. Toss in drained pineapple and mix well then pour it all into a 9x13 inch pan.

6. Refrigerate this mixture for 1 hour.

7. Prepare the snow topping by mixing the ¾ sugar and cream cheese in a mixer.

8. Spread this mixture over the refrigerated cranberry mixture.

9. Serve fresh.

Nutrition

- Calories: 210

- Protein: 2g

- Carbohydrates: 35g

- Fat: 7g

- Cholesterol: 23mg

- Sodium: 58mg

- Potassium: 65mg

- Phosphorus: 25mg

- Calcium: 28mg

- Fiber: 1.0g

183. Berries in Crepes

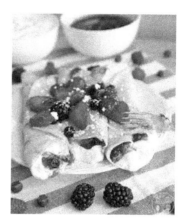

Preparation Time: 15 minutes

Cooking Time: 20 minutes

Servings: 4

Ingredients

- 1/2 cup all-purpose flour

- 1/2 cup almond milk

- 2 egg whites, beaten

- 1 tablespoon vegetable oil

- Cooking spray

- 1/2 cup frozen berries (mix of strawberries, raspberries, blueberries), thawed and drained

- 1 tablespoon powdered sugar

Directions

1. In a bowl, mix the flour, almond milk, egg whites and oil.

2. Spray oil on your pan.

3. Turn the stove to medium heat.

4. Pour 1/4 cup of the flour mixture into the pan.

5. Let the batter spread by moving the pan in a circular motion.

6. Cook until golden.

7. Put the berries on top of the crepe.

8. Let it cook for another 2 minutes before folding the crepe in half.

9. Repeat for the rest of the batter.

10. Sprinkle powdered sugar on top before serving.

Nutrition

- Calories: 124
- Protein: 5g
- Carbohydrates: 17g
- Fat: 4g
- Cholesterol: 0mg
- Sodium: 41mg
- Potassium: 123mg
- Phosphorus: 55mg
- Calcium: 47mg

184. Mini Apple Pies

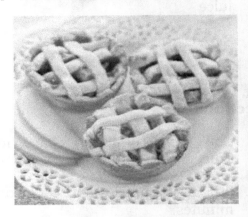

Preparation Time: 20 minutes

Cooking Time: 30 minutes

Servings: 18

Ingredients

- 9-inch single crust pies
- 1½ cups diced Granny Smith apple
- ¼ cup honey
- Lemon juice
- 1/8 teaspoon ground nutmeg
- ¼ teaspoon ground cinnamon

Directions

1. Preheat oven to 400 degrees F.

2. Cut 2 x16-inch rounds out of the pie crusts, and fit them into 2 ×3-inch mini pie dishes.

3. Stir the mixture again, and spoon into the pie shells. Use the strips of dough to weave a small lattice crust on top of each pie, and pinch the strips onto the bottom crust.

4. Bake in the preheated oven until the pies are browned and the filling is thickened and bubbling about 30 minutes. Cool before serving.

Nutrition

- Calories: 114

- Sodium: 4mg

- Protein: 0.2g

- Potassium: 36mg

- Phosphorus: 25mg

185. Gumdrop Cookies

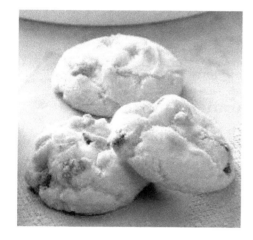

Preparation Time: 15 minutes

Cooking Time: 12 minutes

Servings: 25

Ingredients

- ½ cup of spreadable unsalted butter

- 1 medium egg

- 1 cup of brown sugar

- 1 ⅔ cups of all-purpose flour, sifted

- ¼ cup of milk

- 1 teaspoon vanilla

- 1 teaspoon of baking powder

- 15 large gumdrops, chopped finely

Directions

1. Preheat the oven at 400°F/195°C.

2. Combine the sugar, butter and egg until creamy.

3. Add the milk and vanilla and stir well.

4. Combine the flour with the baking powder in a different bowl. Incorporate to the sugar, butter mixture, and stir.

5. Add the gumdrops and place the mixture in the fridge for half an hour.

6. Drop the dough with tablespoonful into a lightly greased baking or cookie sheet.

7. Bake for 10-12 minutes or until golden brown in color.

Nutrition

- Calories: 102.17kcal

- Carbohydrate: 16.5g

- Protein: 0.86g Sodium: 23.42mg

- Potassium: 45mg

- Phosphorus: 32.15mg

- Dietary Fiber: 0.13g

- Fat: 4g

186. Pineapple Cake

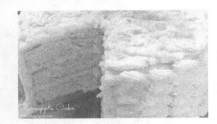

Preparation Time: 15 minutes

Cooking Time: 60 minutes

Servings: 10

Ingredients

- 1 large egg
- ¼ cup olive oil
- 1 cup honey
- 1½ teaspoons vanilla
- 1 pineapple
- 1 cup all-purpose flour
- 1 teaspoon cinnamon
- 1 teaspoon baking soda
- 4 ounces cream cheese

Directions

1. Preheat oven to 350ºF. Spray 9x 13-inch baking pan with non-stick cooking spray. Set cream cheese out to soften. Peel, core and chop pineapples.

2. Mix together eggs oil, honey and vanilla. Stir in pineapples.

3. In a separate bowl, stir together flour, cinnamon, and baking soda.

4. Add dry mixture to pineapple mixture and mix it together.

5. Put into baking pan and bake for one hour. Allow to cool.

Nutrition

- Calories: 254 Sodium: 68mg
- Protein: 3g Potassium: 74mg
- Phosphorus: 20mg

187. Blueberry Crisp

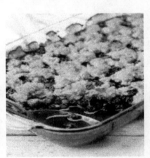

Preparation Time: 15 minutes

Cooking Time: 40 minutes

Servings: 2

Ingredients

- 1 cup fresh blueberries
- 1/8 cup all-purpose flour
- ½ tablespoon honey
- 1/8 teaspoon ground cinnamon
- 1 tablespoon mayonnaise

Directions

1. Preheat the oven to 350 degrees F.

2. Place the blueberries into an 8-inch square baking dish. In a medium bowl, stir together the flour, honey, and cinnamon. Sprinkle over the top of the berries. Bake for 35 to 40 minutes in the preheated oven, until the top is lightly browned.

Nutrition

- Calories: 115 Sodium: 53mg

- Protein: 1.5g Potassium: 68mg

- Phosphorus: 48mg

188. Cherry Crisp

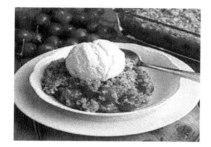

Preparation Time: 15 minutes

Cooking Time: 40 minutes

Servings: 4

Ingredients

- 1 (21 ounces) can cherry pie filling

- ½ cup all-purpose flour

- 2/3 cup honey

- 3/4 teaspoon ground cinnamon

- 3/4 teaspoon ground nutmeg

- 1/3 cup melted butter

Directions

1. Preheat oven to 350 degrees F. Lightly grease a 2-quart baking dish.

2. In a medium bowl, mix together flour, honey, cinnamon, and nutmeg. Mix in melted butter. Spread over pie filling.

3. Bake in the preheated oven for 30 minutes, or until topping is golden brown. Allow to cool 15 minutes before serving.

Nutrition

- Calories: 359 Sodium: 92mg

- Protein: 1.7g Potassium: 140mg

- Phosphorus: 128mg

189. Sweet Cracker Pie Crust

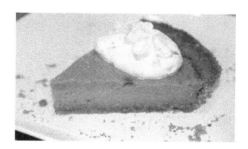

Preparation Time: 15 minutes

Cooking Time: 40 minutes

Servings: 4

Ingredients

- 1 bowl gelatin cracker crumbs

- 1/4 small cup sugar

- Unsalted butter

Direction

- Mix sweet cracker crumbs, butter and sugar. Put in the over preheat at 375°F. Bake for 7 minutes putting it in a greased pie.

- Let the pie cool before adding any kind of filling. Serve and enjoy!

Nutrition

- Calories: 205 Protein: 2g

- Sodium: 208mg Potassium: 67mg

- Phosphorus: 22mg

190. Easy Apple Grits Crisp

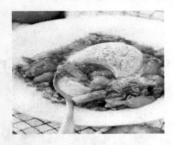

Preparation Time: 30 minutes

Cooking Time: 35 minutes

Servings: 2

Ingredients

- 2 Granny Smith apples

- ¼ cup grits - ¼ cup honey

- 1/8 cup all-purpose flour

- ¼ teaspoon cinnamon

- 1/8 cup butter

Directions

1. Preheat oven to 350°F. Peel, core and slice apples.

2. In a bowl, mix grits, honey, flour and cinnamon.

3. Cut butter into the mixture with a pastry cutter until well blended.

4. Place sliced apples in 9 x 9-inch baking pan.

5. Sprinkle the mixture over apples.

6. Bake for 30 to 35 minutes.

Nutrition

- Calories: 195 Sodium: 64mg

- Protein: 1g Potassium: 138mg

- Phosphorus: 130mg

191. Pound Cake with Pineapple

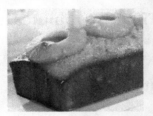

Preparation Time: 10 minutes

Cooking Time: 50 minutes

Servings: 24

Ingredients

- 3 cups of all-purpose flour, sifted

- 3 cups of sugar

- 1 ½ cups of butter

- 6 whole eggs and 3 egg whites

- 1 teaspoon of vanilla extract

- 1 10. Ounce can of pineapple chunks, rinsed and crushed (keep juice aside).

For glaze:

- 1 cup of sugar

- 1 stick of unsalted butter or margarine

- Reserved juice from the pineapple

Directions

1. Preheat the oven at 350°F/180°C.

2. Beat the sugar and the butter with a hand mixer until creamy and smooth.

3. Slowly add the eggs (one or two every time) and stir well after pouring each egg.

4. Add the vanilla extract, follow up with the flour and stir well.

5. Add the drained and chopped pineapple.

6. Pour the mixture into a greased cake tin and bake for 45-50 minutes.

7. In a small saucepan, combine the sugar with the butter and pineapple juice. Stir every few seconds and bring to boil. Cook until you get a creamy to thick glaze consistency.

8. Pour the glaze over the cake while still hot.

9. Let cook for at least 10 seconds and serve.

Nutrition

- Calories: 407.4kcal

- Carbohydrate: 79g

- Protein: 4.25g

- Sodium: 118.97mg

- Potassium: 180.32mg

- Phosphorus: 66.37mg

- Dietary Fiber: 2.25g

- Fat: 16.48g

192. Apple Crunch Pie

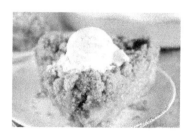

Preparation Time: 10 minutes

Cooking Time: 35 minutes

Servings: 8

Ingredients

- 4 large tart apples, peeled, seeded and sliced

- ½ cup of white all-purpose flour

- ⅓ Cup margarine

- 1 cup of sugar

- ¾ cup of rolled oat flakes

- ½ teaspoon of ground nutmeg

Directions

1. Preheat the oven to 375°F/180°C.

2. Place the apples over a lightly greased square pan (around 7 inches).

3. Mix the rest of the ingredients in a medium bowl with and spread the batter over the apples.

4. Bake for 30-35 minutes or until the top crust has gotten golden brown. Serve hot.

Nutrition

- Calories: 261.9kcal

- Carbohydrate: 47.2g

- Protein: 1.5g Sodium: 81mg

- Potassium: 123.74mg

- Phosphorus: 35.27mg

- Dietary Fiber: 2.81g Fat: 7.99g

193. Chocolate Trifle

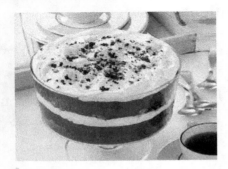

Preparation Time: 10 minutes

Cooking Time: 15 minutes

Servings: 4

Ingredients

- 1 small plain sponge Swiss roll

- 3 oz. custard powder

- 5 oz. hot water

- 16 oz. canned mandarins

- 3 tablespoons sherry

- 5 oz. double cream

- 4 chocolate squares, grated

Directions

1. Whisk the custard powder with water in a bowl until dissolved.

2. In a bowl, mix the custard well until it becomes creamy and let it sit for 15 minutes.

3. Spread the Swiss roll and cut it in 4 squares.

4. Place the Swiss roll in the 4 serving cups.

5. Top the Swiss roll with mandarin, custard, cream, and chocolate.

6. Serve.

Nutrition

- Calories: 315 Sodium: 185mg

- Protein: 2.9g Calcium: 61mg

- Phosphorous: 184mg

- Potassium: 129mg

194. Pineapple Meringues

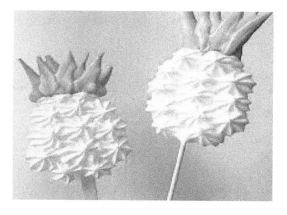

Preparation Time: 10 minutes

Cooking Time: 0 minutes

Servings: 4

Ingredients

- 4 meringue nests
- 8 oz. crème fraiche
- 2 oz. stem ginger, chopped
- 8 oz. can pineapple chunks

Directions

1. Place the meringue nests on the serving plates.
2. Whisk the ginger with crème Fraiche and pineapple chunks.
3. Divide this the pineapple mixture over the meringue nests.
4. Serve.

Nutrition

- Calories: 312
- Sodium: 41mg
- Protein: 2.3g
- Phosphorous: 104mg
- Potassium: 110mg

195. Baked Custard

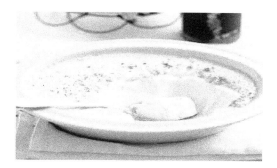

Preparation Time: 10 minutes

Cooking Time: 30 minutes

Servings: 2

Ingredients

- 1/2 cup milk
- 1 egg, beaten
- 1/8 teaspoon nutmeg
- 1/8 teaspoon vanilla
- Sweetener, to taste
- 1/2 cup water

Directions

1. Lightly warm up the milk in a pan, then whisk in the egg, nutmeg, vanilla and sweetener.
2. Pour this custard mixture into a ramekin.

3. Place the ramekin in a baking pan and pour ½ cup water into the pan.

4. Bake the custard for 30 minutes at 325 degrees F.

5. Serve fresh.

Nutrition

- Calories: 127

- Sodium: 119mg

- Protein: 9.6g

- Calcium: 169mg

- Phosphorous: 309mg

- Potassium: 171mg

196. Strawberry Pie

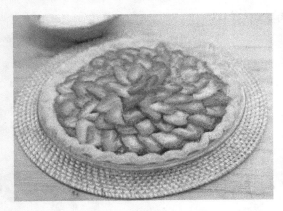

Preparation Time: 10 minutes

Cooking Time: 25 minutes

Servings: 6

Ingredients

- 1 unbaked (9 inches) pie shell

- 4 cups strawberries, fresh

- 1 cup of brown Swerve

- 3 tablespoons arrowroot powder

- 2 tablespoons lemon juice

- 8 tablespoons whipped cream topping

Directions

1. Spread the pie shell in the pie pan and bake it until golden brown.

2. Now mash 2 cups of strawberries with the lemon juice, arrowroot powder, and Swerve in a bowl.

3. Add the mixture to a saucepan and cook on moderate heat until it thickens.

4. Allow the mixture to cool then spread it in the pie shell.

5. Slice the remaining strawberries and spread them over the pie filling.

6. Refrigerate for 1 hour then garnish with whipped cream.

7. Serve fresh and enjoy.

Nutrition

- Calories: 236

- Sodium: 183mg

- Protein: 2.2g

- Calcium: 23mg

- Phosphorous: 47.2mg

- Potassium: 178mg

197. Apple Crisp

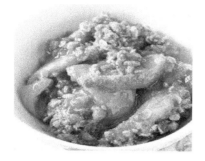

Preparation Time: 10 minutes

Cooking Time: 45 minutes

Servings: 6

Ingredients

- 4 cups apples, peeled and chopped
- ½ teaspoon stevia
- 3 tablespoons brandy
- 2 teaspoons lemon juice
- 1/2 teaspoon cinnamon
- 1/8 teaspoon nutmeg
- 3/4 cup dry oats
- 1/4 cup brown Swerve
- 2 tablespoons flour
- 2 tablespoons butter

Directions

1. Toss the oats with the flour, butter and brown Swerve in a bowl and keep it aside.

2. Whisk the remaining crisp ingredients in an 8-inch baking pan.

3. Spread the oats mixture over the crispy filling.

4. Bake it for 45 minutes at 350 degrees F in a preheated oven.

5. Slice and serve.

Nutrition

- Calories: 214 Sodium: 48mg
- Protein: 2.1g Calcium: 15mg
- Phosphorous: 348mg
- Potassium: 212mg

198. Almond Cookies

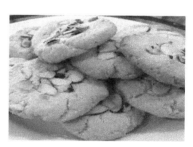

Preparation Time: 10 minutes

Cooking Time: 12 minutes

Servings: 24

Ingredients

- 1 cup butter, softened
- 1 cup granulated Swerve
- 1 egg
- 3 cups flour
- 1 teaspoon baking soda

- 1 teaspoon almond extract

Directions

1. Beat the butter with the Swerve in a mixer then gradually stir in the remaining ingredients.

2. Mix well until it forms a cookie dough then divide the dough into small balls.

3. Spread each ball into ¾ inch rounds and place them in a cookie sheet.

4. Poke 2-3 holes in each cookie then bake for 12 minutes at 400 degrees F.

5. Serve.

Nutrition

- Calories: 159 Sodium: 144mg

- Protein: 1.9g Calcium: 6mg

- Phosphorous: 274mg

- Potassium: 23mg

199. Lime Pie

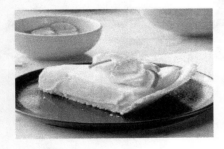

Preparation Time: 5 minutes

Cooking Time: 5 minutes

Servings: 8

Ingredients

- 5 tablespoons butter, unsalted

- 1 1/4 cups breadcrumbs

- 1/4 cup granulated Swerve

- 1/3 cup lime juice

- 14 oz. condensed milk

- 1 cup heavy whipping cream

- 1 (9 inches) pie shell

Directions

1. Switch on your gas oven and preheat it to 350 degrees F. Whisk the cracker crumbs with the Swerve and melted butter in a suitable bowl. Spread this cracker crumbs crust in a 9 inches pie shell and bake it for 5 minutes. Meanwhile, mix the condensed milk with the lime juice in a bowl.

2. Whisk the heavy cream in a mixer until foamy, then add in the condensed milk mixture.

3. Mix well, then spread this filling in the baked crust.

4. Refrigerate the pie for 4 hours.

5. Slice and serve.

Nutrition

- Calories: 391 Sodium: 252mg

- Protein: 5.3g Calcium: 163mg

- Phosphorous: 199mg

- Potassium: 221mg

200. Raspberry Muffins

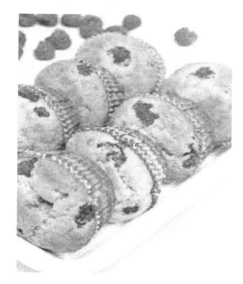

Preparation Time: 10 minutes

Cooking Time: 20 minutes

Servings: 10

Ingredients

- 2 tbsps. Margarine
- 1 ½ tsps. Baking soda
- ½ cup liquid non-dairy creamer
- 2 tsps. Cinnamon
- 1 cup fresh raspberries
- 1 Omega-3 egg
- ¼ cup flour
- ½ cup stevia
- 1 1/3 cups flour
- ¼ cup margarine
- ¼ cup stevia

Directions

1. Preheat your oven to a temperature of 375°F.

2. Line 16 muffin cups with paper liners; then combine about 1 and 1/3 cups of flour with the baking soda in a small bowl and stir in the raspberries

3. In a separate medium bowl; beat the ¼ cup of margarine with the brown sugar and the egg and blender very well

4. Add in the flour and stir until your mixture becomes smooth

5. Spoon the batter in about 16 muffin cups

6. In another bowl, mix the stevia with ¼ cup of flour, 2 tablespoons of margarine and the cinnamon; then sprinkle it over the muffins

7. Bake your muffins for about 15 to 18 minutes

8. Serve and enjoy your muffins!

Nutrition

- Calories: 156.2
- Fat: 10g
- Carbs: 13g
- Potassium: 56mg
- Sodium: 111mg
- Phosphorous: 69g
- Protein: 3g

Conclusion

Prevention of diseases that can affect the kidneys starts at the table. Nutrition plays a fundamental role in ensuring the health of these organs, which perform some essential functions for the body. They allow the elimination of toxins from the blood, instead retaining some vital substances and regulating the volume of the body's liquids, as well as the electrolyte balance.

The kidneys are organs responsible for the filtration of blood, therefore they are essential for human life. In order to guarantee its integrity, it is advisable to recognize and remove the etiological agents that can compromise them; among these: drug abuse, inappropriate food behaviors, alcoholism, sports doping, drug addiction, infections, hypertension, diabetes, and impairment of other organs.

The diet plays a key role in maintaining kidney health; in fact, the scraps of ALL the previously digested-absorbed-metabolized nutritional molecules are filtered by the circulatory stream thanks to the kidney, then collected in the bladder and expelled with urine through urination.

CPSIA information can be obtained
at www.ICGtesting.com
Printed in the USA
LVHW060116150121
676529LV00015B/842